WHAT HAS GOVERNMENT DONE TO OUR HEALTH CARE?

Dr. Charles VanEaton
670 Wright Street
Jonesville, MI 49250

WHAT HAS GOVERNMENT DONE TO OUR HEALTH CARE?

Terree P. Wasley

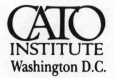

CATO INSTITUTE
Washington D.C.

Library of Congress Cataloging-in-Publication Data

Wasley, Terree P.
  What has government done to our health care? / Terree P. Wasley.
    p. cm.
  Includes bibliographical references and index.
  ISBN 0-932790-88-7 : $19.95.—ISBN 0-932790-87-9 : $10.95
    1. Medicine, State—United States. 2. Medical policy—United
States. 3. Medical care—United States.
    [DNLM: 1. Consumer Satisfaction—United States. 2. Delivery of
Health Care—organization & administration—United
States. 3. Health Services Accessibility—United States. 4. Public
Policy—United States. W 84 AA1 W319w]
  RA395.A3W38 1992
  362.1'0973—dc20
  DNLM/DLC
  for Library of Congress   92-20121
                                                             CIP

ISBN: 0-932790-88-7
ISBN: 0-932790-87-9

Printed in the United States of America.

CATO INSTITUTE
224 Second Street, S.E.
Washington, D.C. 20003

Contents

Preface

The idea that government control of medical care could somehow make it better is not new. As Terree Wasley shows in this superb book, it has been around a long time. The push for a greater government role in medical care varies in intensity with the political climate. When the pressure is more intense I am occasionally asked, usually on some social occasion, "Tell me, doctor, how do you feel about socialized medicine?" Whether the questioner sincerely wants my opinion or just wants to argue, my answer is always the same, "I have only one real worry about it: What is going to happen to my family or me when we become patients?" That leads to a productive discussion with those who are really interested and effectively quiets those who are merely argumentative.

Now that government actions directly or indirectly determine what happens with health care in this country and I'm eligible to be a Medicare beneficiary, my old worry is becoming a sad reality. Because I had been in practice for 19 years before Medicare took effect in 1966, I have had a standard by which to evaluate the changes that have occurred since the government became involved in a big way. The results have been much worse than anything I imagined.

When I get sick, I want to be able to choose my own physician. That essential freedom is being denied to many patients who belong to managed (that is, rationed) care programs. The ability of Medicare patients to see the doctor of their choice will soon be impaired as well because of a ridiculous requirement that all physicians be paid the same for each service they perform. Thus, a highly qualified specialist who is in great demand will be paid no more than a physician who is barely qualified. It's as though Michael Jordan were paid no more for playing basketball than a rookie who spends 95 percent of his time on the bench. Medicare patients are not allowed to pay more than the government-set amount even if they want to and can easily afford to. Obviously, such price controls will make it less desirable for top physicians to see Medicare patients. So the medical care of elderly citizens will deteriorate.

We now find ourselves in a bizarre situation. Modern science has given us an unsurpassed capability to prevent, diagnose, and treat disease, but barriers prevent many Americans from getting the potential benefits of that care. Those barriers result from misguided efforts to control costs that were caused by government regulations, excessive utilization of services due to illogical insurance reimbursement policies, and claims for malpractice. The inevitable result will be that Americans will suffer needlessly and die when they shouldn't.

The media deluge us with the perceived problems of our health care system. Curiously, the people who are the most vociferous in pointing out the failures of previous government programs are the ones pushing for even more government control to somehow solve the problems those very government actions have caused. We might look on them as government-control addicts who crave more and more of the drug that is destroying them. The lack of understanding of the true nature of health care problems on the part of physicians and other health care professionals, as well as the general public and the advocates of government control, is truly impressive and depressing.

In this excellent book, Terree Wasley explains in a clear and readable manner how we got into the present mess. She presents a fine brief history of medical regulation, with special attention to the unintended perverse consequences of that regulation. Her analysis shows that without a doubt, the fundamental flaw in the system is lack of consumer power over and responsibility for spending on medical care. She then demolishes the current proposals for further government control of medical care and reviews the government programs that have been tried in other countries. She ably strips away the mystique of the Canadian system that has caught the fancy of many Americans and shows that the United States should not emulate it. Finally, she outlines what we need to do to restore to ourselves control over our health care. Her proposals include measures to remove government distortion of the insurance industry and the creation of tax-free medical savings accounts to let people take charge of their own spending on medical care.

Anyone interested in what ails the health care system in America—not just those of us working in the field but all of us as potential patients—will profit from reading this book. In the coming debate over health care reform, I sincerely hope that the ideas in Terree Wasley's book get a wide hearing.

PHILLIPS L. GAUSEWITZ, M.D.

Acknowledgments

The United States stands at a crossroads. In many areas of public policy the achievements of past programs are being reevaluated. The health care system is no exception, and the citizens of this nation will soon face significant choices regarding the direction of any reform. Realizing that the public needs and wants to make informed decisions on issues, I wrote this book in an attempt to provide a glimpse at history and the errors that were made. I hope it encourages the development of a health care system that corrects any mistakes and allows everyone access at an affordable price.

I wish to thank Ed Crane, president of the Cato Institute, for allowing me the opportunity to write this book, and the staff at Cato for their assistance in its publication. I would also express my appreciation to Dr. Phillips Gausewitz for his direction and advice. A special thank you goes to Congressman Jon Kyl and two members of his staff, Tammy Weinbrenner and Cindi Berry, who were always prompt in providing information and assistance.

I would specifically like to acknowledge those authors whose works provided invaluable material used throughout this book, namely, Paul Starr, author of *The Social Transformation of American Medicine;* Stuart M. Butler and Edward F. Haislmaier, *Critical Issues: A National Health System for America;* and John C. Goodman and Gerald L. Musgrave. Their contributions to our understanding of the health care system should not be underestimated.

I would be remiss if I did not recognize all the physicians and patients I interviewed across this country. Their experiences with the health care system, whether as practitioners or participants, were invaluable.

Finally, I wish to thank my entire family, especially Jeff and Caitlin, for their unlimited patience and support. I dedicate this book to Caitlin, for she will live most of her life under whatever kind of health care system we ultimately choose.

1. Introduction

Kate and Joe have been married 17 years.[1] Joe has an excellent job with a good company, and Kate works at home with their two children—Kenny, age nine, and Annie, age five. They live in a comfortable house in the suburbs of St. Louis, Missouri. They are a happy family, but there is one thing that concerns Joe and Kate. Because something beyond their control happened to their family five years ago, they are now entangled in a web woven by their health insurance.

You see, Annie was born with cerebral palsy and needs extensive and costly medical care. Joe's company provides good health care benefits that cover most of Annie's medical needs. Joe likes his job very much, but he realizes his future mobility is severely restricted. He cannot change his job or career without risking the loss of insurance coverage for Annie because of her preexisting condition. And Joe and Kate, like most other people, could not afford that loss. So they will most likely remain in the St. Louis area, in their house in the suburbs, for a long, long time—whether they want to or not.

Jeff and Cindy are newlyweds, living in a small town on the outskirts of Washington, D.C. He is a self-employed contractor, and she teaches dance at the local studio. While Cindy was working for the public schools as a teacher, she had Blue Cross/Blue Shield health coverage. Her insurance served her well when she was diagnosed as having Graves' disease, a thyroid condition, a few months before her wedding. The hospital and medical costs were expensive, but the insurance paid for most of them. When Cindy stopped teaching, however, the insurance eventually ran out. Jeff and Cindy recently applied for health insurance for themselves, but they were turned down. The reason, the insurance company told

---

[1]The stories in this introduction are true, but the names of the individuals have been changed. Throughout this book, however, physicians and other medical personnel are identified by their real names.

1

Cindy, was that she has a preexisting condition. Currently, she and Jeff have no health insurance.

Dr. Paul Glanville of Chandler, Arizona, calls himself "the new, improved horse-and-buggy doctor." In 1988, when the cost of his malpractice premium soared to more than he could afford, he dropped the insurance. Canceling it meant that he also had to drop all his health maintenance organization (HMO) and preferred provider organization (PPO) programs. Soon he discovered that those programs had contributed 70 percent of his gross business income, so he said goodbye to his nurse and secretary. He gave his patients their medical charts and told them to bring their records in when they came to see him.

His old practice required an overhead of about $14,000 a month. He had a business consultant, a new computer system to handle all the HMO and PPO paperwork, a secretary, and one nurse. Now his overhead is approximately $1,200 a month, his gross personal income is $42,000 a year, he takes 12 weeks vacation, and he charges his patients $10 per visit. Glanville has challenged medical convention: "If enough doctors would leave the system and become radical, how much could we trim from costs? Would ordinary working people then be able to afford insurance again?"[2]

Health care costs and coverage have become a dominant force in almost everyone's life over the course of the last 50 years. One of the first questions young people entering the job market are taught to ask is, "What are the benefits with this job?" Before many workers change jobs, they must weigh the costs of changes in health coverage. Many people are left out of the insurance market because they can't get coverage, can't afford it, or make too much money to be covered by a government program.

Patients complain that some doctors don't listen anymore, and they are anxious to slap their physician with a lawsuit for the slightest imperfection in care. Physicians are tired of struggling under the mountains of paperwork required by the government and insurance companies, when all they want to do is treat patients.

And costs keep going up. With 1992 health care expenditures expected to reach $832 billion, the American public wonders where

[2]Condensed from "The New, Improved Horse-and-Buggy Doctor," *AAPS News* 46, no. 6 (June 1990): 2.

all the money is going.[3] Many remember the good old days when costs were lower, coverage was better, and paperwork wasn't so complicated. Fingers are pointed at shady insurance companies, greedy doctors, and wasteful government. No one can figure out the answer. All that anyone knows is that costs are too high and too many people are falling through the cracks of the health care system.

How have we in the United States gotten into this mess? Why are some people shut out of the health insurance market and others trapped in lives that they may or may not want but cannot change because of their health insurance? Why are some physicians forced to quit, take early retirement, or radically alter their practices? What has caused health care costs to careen out of control? Should we throw up our hands, as have some of the experts, and resign ourselves to a system of nationalized health care as our only option?

Why am I writing a book on the health care crisis? Because the cost of providing health care services to the American people has risen to the point where those who are insured are concerned for people who are not. The number of uninsured is on the rise, with estimates ranging from 31 million to 37 million.[4] According to a 1991 *Wall Street Journal*/NBC News poll, 32 percent of those responding said that people not covered by any health insurance constituted the most important health care issue facing the country.[5]

Dissatisfaction with the current state of health care has bred disdain for the U.S. system and has been accompanied by accusations that a free market in health care has failed. Such critical reaction has focused attention on proposals for national health care, which some see as the only solution to the problems of the uninsured and rising costs. Others promote increased reliance on market processes to solve the health care dilemma, and those people point to the collapse of government-run systems all over the world as proof that government cannot solve the problem.

---

[3]Data from personal interview with Sharon Silow-Carroll of New Directions for Policy, Washington, D.C.

[4]U.S. Bureau of the Census, *Current Population Survey*, March 1990.

[5]Michel McQueen, "Voters, Sick of the Current Health-Care System, Want Federal Government to Prescribe Remedy," *Wall Street Journal*, June 28, 1991. Fifty-five percent said the "high cost of health care" was the most important issue.

This book has been written especially for those who are not health care experts but who use the health care system—and that ultimately includes all of us. Chapter 2 takes a close look at what both providers and receivers of health care are saying. It covers some of the problems, difficulties, and frustrations that face doctors, nurses, and hospital administrators today. And it looks at the current concerns of patients and their complaints about the system they use to keep healthy.

Following an examination of what troubles and pleases both sides, Chapter 3 provides a history of the development of the health care industry in the 20th century, as well as explanations and an analysis of how we arrived at our present state.

Chapter 4 includes a detailed investigation of some of the proposed solutions to our current problems that would take us in the direction of a national system of health care. Proposals to adopt a Canadian-style program are discussed, as are the opinions of some people that other proposals and processes already under way are sending us into a gradual slide toward national health care. This chapter also includes an explanation and analysis of some of the European, British, and Canadian health care systems and whether or not they would provide a workable solution for the United States.

Chapter 5 examines reforms of the health care system that would provide individuals greater freedom of choice in health care. Emphasis is placed on greater control by the individual over his health care, expanded access to health care and insurance coverage for those currently shut out of the market, and increased options for high-quality health care for the poor and elderly. The ultimate goal of such reforms is to expand access to the health care system to all by concurrently lowering the costs of health care and providing the greatest number of choices to individuals at all income levels.

2. The Reality of 20th-Century Health Care

Most Americans think of their health care system in the same way that they think of Congress. In recent years the American public has displayed increasing displeasure with the way Congress operates. Poll after poll has revealed rising disgust with members of Congress in the management of their personal affairs and distrust of their handling of the affairs of government. The cry of "Throw the bums out" is heard throughout the land, and incumbents' losing their jobs on a massive scale is discussed almost daily in the national media.

In spite of all this displeasure (as the election results showed in 1990), an overwhelming number of incumbents continue to be reelected to Congress.[1] And a peculiar phenomenon occurs when citizens are asked not about Congress in general but about their own representatives. Most people support their representative and think that he or she is doing a good job for their state. It's always the other members of Congress who need to be replaced.

The Patients

Americans appear to be as schizophrenic about their health care as they are about Congress. A 1986 survey showed that 75 percent of the public believed that the U.S. health care system required fundamental change.[2] By November 1991, according to a recent *Time*/CNN poll, that proportion had risen to 91 percent.[3] On the other hand, according to the 1986 survey, approximately 75 percent

---

[1]Ninety-six percent of House incumbents seeking reelection were successful in the November 1990 elections. "Election Ferment" (editorial), *Wall Street Journal*, November 8, 1990.

[2]Carl J. Schramm, ed., *Health Care and Its Costs* (New York: W. W. Norton & Company, 1987), 53.

[3]Janet Castro, "Ten Ways to Cure the Health Care Mess," *Time*, November 25, 1991, p. 34.

of those who had actually been hospitalized in the previous year and more than 80 percent of those who had seen a physician recently were completely satisfied with the medical care they had received.[4]

The Doctor-Patient Relationship

This finding was also seen in a 1990 Gallup poll in Arizona, in which 65 percent of Arizonans said they were very satisfied with their primary-care physician.[5] According to a 1990 survey of public opinion conducted by the American Medical Association (AMA), 85 percent of those surveyed said that, overall, they were very satisfied with their last visit to the doctor, 90 percent were pleased with the way they had been treated, and 85 percent were satisfied with the medical care they had received.[6]

In a 1991 *Fortune* poll, 95 percent of corporate executive officers said they were satisfied with the quality of health care their employees received.[7] And 98 percent of those responding to a 1990 patient attitude survey conducted for *Medical Economics* rated their physician's staff as competent or extremely competent, and 82 percent considered the assistants courteous.[8]

In the *Medical Economics* survey, 86 percent of the respondents reported that their physicians spent enough time with them. Of those polled in a 1986 survey, 80 percent had positive feelings

[4]Carl J. Schramm; *Special Report: Access to Health Care in the United States: Results of a 1986 Survey*, no. 2 (Princeton, N.J.: Robert Wood Foundation, 1987).

[5]David Cannella, "Arizonans Polled on Health Care," *Arizona Republic*, November 8, 1990.

[6]American Medical Association, *Surveys of Physician and Public Opinion on Health Care Issues* (1990)—hereinafter the AMA opinion surveys. The data reported for physicians were the result of nationwide telephone interviews with 1,009 physicians, 49 percent of whom were members of the AMA and 51 percent of whom were nonmembers. The public opinion portion was based on telephone interviews with 1,500 randomly selected U.S. residents aged 18 or older. The AMA commissioned the Gallup Organization to perform the study.

[7]William E. Sheeline, "Taking on Public Enemy No. 1," *Fortune*, July 1, 1991.

[8]Results of the entire survey were incorporated into a series of four articles in the April 23, 1990, edition of *Medical Economics*. These particular data came from Mark Crane, "Your Office: Making Things Easier for Patients Pays Off," *Medical Economics*, April 23, 1990, p. 63. This survey—hereinafter the *Medical Economics* survey—was conducted by National Family Opinion, Inc. More than 1,050 people answered the eight-page survey's detailed questions about their relationship with their physician and their feelings about the health care system.

toward their doctor.[9] When I asked patients if they were pleased with their relationship with their doctor, an overwhelming majority said they liked—and had a positive relationship with—their physician.

The Increasing Cost of Health Care

Although 75 percent of people in a 1991 poll said that health care costs were much higher than they should have been,[10] many patients say that they are not significantly affected by the increased costs of medical care. That is because most citizens have been shielded from the cost of care by a third party (private or government insurance) and have been insulated from the meteoric rise in costs. The proportion of the population with health insurance has remained between 86 and 87 percent in recent years.[11] The Health Insurance Association of America estimates that more than 181 million Americans have one or more forms of private insurance protection.[12] In the *Medical Economics* survey, 53 percent of those responding had traditional insurance, such as Blue Cross/Blue Shield; 25 percent were covered under Medicare; 18 percent were covered by an HMO or a PPO; and 7 percent had no insurance.

The majority of patients I spoke with were covered by some form of insurance, either private or government provided. Many commented that because of their insurance they really didn't pay too much attention to the actual cost of their care. A music teacher in Illinois remarked that her family "noticed the higher costs but kept going anyway." In Washington, D.C., a manager commented, "I have an HMO through my company so we don't notice the higher costs."

Third-party insurance (whether private, Medicare, Medicaid, or another government program) pays more than 73 percent of the

[9]Schramm, *Special Report.*

[10]1991 *Time/*CNN poll.

[11]Charles Nelson and Kathleen Short, *Health Insurance Coverage 1986–1988, Survey of Income and Program Participation* (U.S. Bureau of the Census, 1990).

[12]American College of Physicians, "Access to Health Care" (position paper), *Annals of Internal Medicine* 112, no. 9 (May 1, 1990).

health care bills in the United States.[13] The federal and state governments now cover 42 cents of every dollar spent on health care.[14]

Some people do complain about higher medical costs, and they usually are those who are self-employed or own small businesses. A farmer in Nebraska, for example, complained that "doctor calls are expensive, so we don't go very often," and a Maryland businessman stated that "our family will need to change insurance soon due to the high cost of premiums." However, according to the 1990 AMA surveys, only 15 percent of those interviewed said that they had not sought medical treatment because the cost for the service was too high. On the other hand, 84 percent of those responding to the *Medical Economics* survey said they had *never* had to postpone or cancel a doctor's appointment because they couldn't afford to pay for it.

Only within the past decade have costs risen to such a high level that some who previously could afford coverage now find health insurance premiums out of their reach. Those who are the most dissatisfied with the current system are the ones forced to forgo insurance—some small business owners and their employees, many of the self-employed, the very poor, and the very sick. The following instance was cited by the *Wall Street Journal*.

> A battle with colon cancer last year was trauma enough for John K. Keitt, president of a Naples, Florida, cabinetwork business. It took $45,000 worth of surgery and care to gain the upper hand. But last summer, Mr. Keitt received another shock: As a result of his illness, the health-insurance bill for his 13-employee business was rising to $56,000 a year from $20,000.
>
> "I was so angry I threw the bill out," he says. "The increase alone would have amounted to 10% of our total overhead costs." Finally, Mr. Keitt found another insurer with affordable premiums—but reduced benefits. He says he mightn't even have gotten that if he hadn't recovered. "If I hadn't beaten cancer, who knows what would have happened?" he asks.[15]

[13]Kathryn M. Welling, "The Sickening Spiral: Health-Care Costs Continue to Grow at an Alarming Rate," *Barron's*, June 11, 1990.

[14]"American Survey: Worrying about Health," *The Economist*, June 15, 1991, p. 27.

[15]Roger Ricklefs, "Health Insurance Becomes a Big Pain for Small Firms," *Wall Street Journal*, December 6, 1989.

Dramatically rising insurance rates were ranked as the number one problem for small business employers and the self-employed, according to a 1989 survey by the National Federation of Independent Business.[16] Small businesses often pay premiums that are 30 to 40 percent higher than those paid by larger firms. Many small companies are finding that they have to cut back or even eliminate coverage for employees because of soaring costs. The cost of providing benefits for a tire retail business in Mauldin, South Carolina, for example, rose from $55,000 to $97,000 from 1988 to 1990. The owner reported that "in the future, we will not be able to provide this benefit for our employees."[17]

According to the Health Insurance Association of America, annual increases in business spending on insurance premiums have been in double digits for the last few years.[18] Nearly one-third of those responding to a 1990 health care survey in *Nation's Business* reported that their health insurance premiums had increased 30 percent or more, and just over one-third of them described increases ranging from 16 percent to 29 percent.[19] In 1989, *D & B Reports* noted that 39 percent of small businesses surveyed had had premium increases of 20 percent or more during 1988—including 9 percent that had had increases of 50 percent or more.[20]

A U.S. Chamber of Commerce survey of almost 1,000 companies found that health-related benefits per employee increased from 8 percent of payroll, or $2,189, in 1987 to 9.3 percent, or $2,853, in 1989—an increase of almost 12 percent per year.[21] According to a survey by A. Foster Higgins and Company, medical plan costs per employee rose to $3,161 in 1990, an increase of 11 percent over the 1989 figure of $2,853.[22]

[16]Ibid.

[17]Small Business USA, "Member Survey Results: Access to Health Care" (Washington: National Small Business United, May/June 1990), p. 7.

[18]Jack Meyer, Sean Sullivan, and Sharon Silow-Carroll, *Critical Choices: Confronting the Cost of American Health Care*, a report by New Directions for Policy for the National Committee for Quality Health Care (Washington, 1990), p. 32.

[19]Roger Thompson, "10 Ways to Cut Your Health-Care Costs Now," *Nation's Business*, October 1990.

[20]Cited in Ricklefs.

[21]Meyer, Sullivan, and Silow-Carroll, p. 32.

[22]Ron Winslow, "Costs of Medical Care Continue to Soar, Defying Corporate Efforts to Find Cures," *Wall Street Journal*, January 29, 1991.

WHAT HAS GOVERNMENT DONE TO OUR HEALTH CARE?

According to an account published in *Fortune* in 1988, Kina Taylor was a typical four-year-old growing up in New Orleans, Louisiana. Her mother, Wendy, age 19, had worked for almost three years serving chicken at a fast-food franchise for $3.45 an hour. The boss provided no health insurance for her or Kina, who suffered from chronic asthma. When Kina had an asthma attack, Wendy would rush her to the emergency room at New Orleans' Charity Hospital for treatment. In an ironic and inequitable twist of fate, although Wendy had no insurance, she was buying insurance for someone else. Of every $100 she earned, the payroll tax nicked her $1.45, and her boss a matching amount, to provide Medicare for today's elderly. In 46 years from 1988, Wendy too will be eligible, assuming that Medicare is still solvent.[23]

Business owners responding to a 1991 National Small Business United survey cited costs as the main reason they did not provide any health benefits (11 percent) or offered benefits to less than 40 percent of their employees (10 percent).[24] Over one-third of the survey respondents said they had employees with preexisting conditions that were excluded from coverage, and 21 percent of them said they had been denied coverage by at least one insurance company.

Job Mobility and Health Insurance

The lack of job mobility, or "job lock" as it is sometimes called, has become an issue when dealing with health insurance. A majority of workers obtain their insurance through their employer or their spouse's employer. A growing number are finding that if they change jobs, they risk losing their health insurance or at least must choose a plan with less-desirable coverage. Restrictions on job mobility were a significant problem for some of the workers I talked with, such as Joe and Kate in the St. Louis area. Those with family members with preexisting conditions can feel trapped in their current jobs, fearing the loss of health insurance. An engineer in Tennessee remarked that he examines the benefits of any new job carefully before changing.

---

[23]Condensed from Lee Smith, "The Battle over Health Insurance," *Fortune*, September 26, 1988, p. 145.

[24]Small Business USA, p. 7.

A switch in jobs often brings new insurance company coverage, forcing many patients to change their family physician. According to the 1990 AMA opinion surveys, 20 percent of those interviewed had been forced to transfer to another physician because of a change in health insurance coverage. Those most likely to experience a change in physicians were aged 35 to 39.

Patients and Physicians: What Caused the Rise in Health Care Costs and What Are the Solutions?

Patients and physicians list a variety of factors as contributing to the escalation in health care costs. Among those most frequently mentioned are malpractice lawsuits and awards; the practice of defensive medicine; interference by third parties, including insurance companies and government; the cost of government health care programs; the proliferation of high-technology equipment; and the high expectations of patients.

Patients and doctors consider malpractice costs a significant contributor to increased health care costs. They are very concerned about the rise in malpractice suits and the need for reform in this area. Both are interested in reducing the number of lawsuits and limiting the amount of awards. Of the corporate, government, and health care leaders interviewed in a Metropolitan Life survey, 84 percent said that they would accept limits on the right to sue for medical malpractice.[25] In the *Medical Economics* survey, 73 percent of patients said they would like to limit lawyers' fees in malpractice cases. What is more, 68 percent favored limits on the size of malpractice awards, 52 percent backed mandatory pretrial screening of liability claims, and 51 percent were ready to restrict the circumstances under which patients could sue their doctors. Dr. John Koch, an otolaryngologist at Johns Hopkins Hospital, remarked, "Tort reform is needed to eliminate the drain on available funds that should go to reimburse patients but instead [go] to legal counsel."[26]

---

[25]This survey, "Trade-offs & Choices: Health Policy Options for the 1990s"—hereinafter the Met Life Survey—was conducted in 1990 for Metropolitan Life Insurance Company by Louis Harris and Associates, New York. It was based on interviews with 2,048 respondents from nine groups, including federal legislators, legislative committee staff, federal regulators, state health care officials, hospital chief executive officers, physician leaders, union leaders, and health insurers.

[26]From correspondence with the author.

WHAT HAS GOVERNMENT DONE TO OUR HEALTH CARE?

To protect themselves from lawsuits, physicians order magnetic resonance imaging scans, blood tests, and myriad other procedures even when they are only remotely relevant. The concern of doctors and patients for defensive medicine is not unwarranted; the AMA estimates that defensive medicine costs $15 billion a year.[27] The *Fortune* poll found that 52 percent of chief executive officers identified unnecessary medical procedures as a primary cause of the rise in health care costs. Asked how often they found themselves practicing defensive medicine, 42 percent of physicians responding to a *Washingtonian* survey answered "frequently," and 35 percent answered "occasionally."[28] More than half said that such measures added as much as 30 percent to their patients' bills. Dr. Paul Parsons, an orthopedic surgeon in Tennessee, commented, "Enacting tort reform, limiting awards, and reducing malpractice premiums will decrease the need for defensive medicine by making suits for all but obvious negligence a thing of the past."[29]

Doctors and patients are also bothered by the detrimental effects of third-party insurance, including government programs such as Medicare and Medicaid. Physicians believe that the lack of patient responsibility and indifference to the cost of care as a result of low deductibles and copayments contribute to overuse of the system, thereby driving up costs. Dr. John Toth, a general practitioner in California, said he believes that patients too often expect someone else to pay for care.[30] Some patients I spoke with, although they liked the idea of complete coverage, were suspicious of its contributions to higher overall health care costs.

Most doctors are unhappy with third-party and government insurance because of the bureaucratic hassles involved, as well as the higher costs. The 1990 AMA opinion surveys reported that 24 percent of doctors believed that third-party payers and paperwork were the most difficult problems in their day-to-day practice. In the 1991 *Washingtonian* survey, 58 percent of doctors said that red tape from insurers is the biggest impediment to their ability to dispense

---

[27]Lee Smith, "A Cure for What Ails Medical Care," *Fortune*, July 1, 1991.

[28]"1991 Washingtonian Physicians Survey," *Washingtonian*, November 1991—hereinafter the *Washingtonian* survey. It was completed by 825 doctors in the Washington and Baltimore area.

[29]From correspondence with the author.

[30]From correspondence with the author.

12

good medical care. More than one-third gave government interference top billing as a primary cause of cost increases. Dr. Stephen Hershey, an orthopedist practicing in Delaware, blamed the rising cost of health care directly on government programs such as Medicare and Medicaid.[31]

Patients and physicians like the availability of high-technology equipment but are concerned about its overuse contributing to higher health care costs. Of the chief executive officers surveyed in the *Fortune* poll, 59 percent cited expensive new technology as a leading cost culprit. Don Parlett, a former associate general manager for an Arizona utility who had handled health care benefits plans for several thousand employees, offered an observation: "The duplication of technological facilities by local hospitals is partly to blame for the rise in costs."[32] In the 1990 AMA opinion surveys, fully three-fourths of physicians said that some kind of cost-benefit analysis should be conducted before reimbursement is approved for new technologies. And in the *Washingtonian* survey, 34 percent of physicians cited the high cost of technology as a major problem with the health care system.

Some physicians believe that many patients' high expectations contribute to rising costs. Consumers of health care services in the United States expect a quick and accurate fix for almost any health problem, and they are inclined to sue if a complete recovery does not happen. As Dr. Alan R. Hudson, president of the Toronto Hospital, has explained, "When an American hits his head on the road, he expects a neurosurgeon to be standing there."[33] Of the physicians responding to the *Washingtonian* survey, 20 percent listed "unreasonable patient expectations" as one of the major impediments to supplying good care. And Kenneth Abramowitz, a medical consultant for Sanford C. Bernstein & Co., observed, "As soon as it's our lives on the line, we want the best health care money can buy."[34]

Physicians are concerned about the poor and their access to high-quality health care. In the 1990 AMA opinion surveys, 88 percent

[31]From correspondence with the author.
[32]From correspondence with the author.
[33]Smith.
[34]Welling.

of physicians said they believed they had an obligation to provide charity care. Dr. Thomas Hartley, an allergist practicing in Arizona, although supportive of a free-market approach, said that doctors should either be required or volunteer to treat indigent patients.[35]

Physicians do provide uncompensated care, amounting to $10.2 billion in 1989.[36] Totally free care provided by physicians amounted to $2.9 billion in 1989. Free care plus reduced-fee care totaled $6.6 billion. Adding the amount written off for bad debts brings the total to $10.2 billion. The proportion of physicians providing charity care rose to 66 percent in 1989 from 62 percent in 1988. Physicians providing such care spend an average of 2.7 hours per week providing free care and 3.5 hours per week providing reduced-fee care. Combined, these figures represented an average of 10 percent of the charity care provider's total hours.

The American public is concerned about those who cannot afford health care services, and polls show that many believe everyone should have equal access to health care regardless of ability to pay.[37] A national Gallup poll conducted for Blue Cross/Blue Shield in July 1990 indicated that 49 percent of those surveyed believed that the federal government should provide health care for everybody.[38] Sixty-six percent of those in the *Time*/CNN poll said that health care was a right. In spite of this willingness to help, however, research done by Dr. Robert Blendon of Harvard University's School of Public Health showed that 75 percent of Americans were unwilling to pay more than $50 a year to provide health care for those falling through the gaps in the current system.[39]

---

[35]From correspondence with the author.

[36]Estimates on uncompensated care are from the AMA's Socioeconomic Monitoring System 1990 core and autumn surveys, provided in correspondence from Lynn Jensen of the AMA, and from the 1989 Physician Masterfile, *Physician Characteristics and Distribution* (Chicago: AMA, Department of Physician Data Services, Division of Survey and Data Resources, 1990).

[37]Sam Hanna, "Americans Want Equal Care for All," *Health Care Competition Week*, January 12, 1987, pp. 3–4; and "Making Difficult Health Care Decisions," a National Public Opinion Survey conducted by Louis Harris and Associates for the Harvard Community Health Plan Foundation, April/May 1987, p. 8.

[38]Beverly Orndorff and Estele Jackson, "Pervasive Hesitancy Keeping Patient Sick," *Richmond Times-Dispatch*, November 22, 1990.

[39]Carol Stevens, "Patients Give Uncle Sam a Big Vote," *Medical Economics*, April 23, 1990, p. 83.

Patients and Physicians: What about National Health Insurance?

The results of polls on national health care are mixed, and some-times contradictory, depending on how the question is posed and who is doing the survey.[40] Most polls show that a significant seg-ment of the public does not have a clear understanding of how a national health care system actually operates. Many polls show a majority of the public to be in favor of some sort of national health insurance plan,[41] while others tell a different story.[42] One thing does seem certain: whenever a price tag is attached to polling questions, support for national health insurance diminishes.

A poll done for the AMA by the Gallup organization in January 1991 showed that 31 percent of those responding supported national health care. But when asked how much they would be willing to pay for it, the majority said no more than $100 a year.[43] An article published in a 1990 issue of the *New England Journal of Medicine* stated that although the majority of Americans said they favored equal access to health care without regard to ability to pay, only 22 percent indicated a willingness to pay more than $200 per year for a universal health plan.[44]

The public does register its dislike for many of the features nor-mally found in national health care plans, such as rationing, waiting

[40]In a Pennsylvania poll conducted following the 1991 Senate election, for example, 60 percent of the recipients said their preference was for the health care system to be run privately. In answer to a subsequent question, however, 60 percent said they favored a Canadian-style system run by the government. "Pennsylvania Post-Election Study," conducted for the Health Insurance Association of America by Public Opinion Strategies and Mellman & Lazrus, November 6–7, 1991.

[41]A 1988 poll conducted by Louis Harris and Dr. Robert Blendon, chairman of the Department of Health Policy and Management at Harvard University's School of Public Health, found that 61 percent of Americans would prefer a system of national health insurance like the one in Canada. A January 1990 poll conducted by the *Los Angeles Times* reported that 66 percent favor a comprehensive national health insurance plan. Both polls are cited in "The Crisis in Health Insurance: Part 2," *Consumer Reports*, September 1990.

[42]Orndorff and Jackson. The July 1990 Gallup/Blue Cross/Blue Shield poll recorded that 43 percent of those surveyed said that a federally financed national health program would be a mistake.

[43]Kevin Anderson, "Taxes May Erode Support for National Health Care," *USA Today*, March 25, 1991.

[44]Robert J. Blendon and Karen Donelan, "Special Report: The Public and the Emerging Debate over National Health Insurance," *New England Journal of Medicine* 323 (July 19, 1990): 208–12.

15

lines, and limits on physician choice.[45] Although most Americans want a health care system that offers equal access and quality for all, they do not want to sacrifice the high quality of care they have become accustomed to. Dr. Richard Bruehlman, a family practitioner in Pennsylvania, said he believes that Americans "would not tolerate for long the decreased quality under [national health insurance]."[46]

Sixty-five percent of physicians responding to the *Washingtonian* survey said they believed that the United States would eventually adopt a national health care system. However, in the Met Life survey, a majority (63 percent) of the leaders of medical societies interviewed said they would not be willing to accept a national health plan even if it guaranteed payment of fees and substantially reduced utilization review, malpractice insurance premiums, and paperwork.

The Met Life survey asked approximately 2,000 business, union, and government leaders if they thought things would get better if the government took over management of the health care system. An overwhelming 79 percent said the situation would not get better, while only 20 percent said it would. The only group believing that things would get better was the union leaders (58 to 38 percent). In addition, 72 percent of those surveyed said they believed that changing to a government health program would increase health care costs, and only 24 percent felt that costs would decrease. By a slight margin (48 to 46 percent), union leaders also said they believed costs would increase.

In a 1990 survey of executives for the Health Insurance Association of America, 94 percent opposed nationalization of health insurance, and 60 percent said that the private sector should take the responsibility for solving the health care financing crisis.[47]

[45]In the Pennsylvania poll cited in footnote 40, 60 percent favored a Canadian-style system. When asked if they would still support such a system if it included waiting times and less access to high technology, 50 percent opposed a nationalized system. The report in the *New England Journal of Medicine* (Blendon and Donelan) said that even though a majority of those polled would support national health insurance, most would not want it if it meant that their freedom of choice of physicians would be limited or if it led to longer waiting times than they now experience.

[46]From correspondence with the author.

[47]Cited in Roger Thompson, "A No to National Health Insurance," *Nation's Business*, May 1990.

16

The Health Care Professionals

Doctors and nurses have a number of complaints about the current health-care situation: bureaucracy, paperwork, the threat of malpractice suits, and especially the impact of such problems on the doctor-patient relationship. More and more doctors are threatening to escape through early retirement.

Mountains of Paperwork

"Physicians spend more time responding to rules, regulations and paper work than I sometimes think they spend caring for patients," complains James Todd, executive director of the AMA.[48] Physicians and their office staffs have become increasingly dissatisfied with the amount of paperwork that is required by a multitude of government and private third-party payers, each with its own rules and requirements for obtaining payment.

The amount of paperwork involved in recording, billing, reviewing, auditing, justifying, and explaining medical charges is tremendous, and it is intruding on physician and staff time available for patient care. In the AMA opinion surveys, 12 percent of doctors said that paperwork and bureaucracy were the most difficult problem they faced in their day-to-day practice of medicine. Another 12 percent stated that third-party payers and reimbursement headaches were their most difficult problem, 11 percent cited intrusion into their practices by outside parties, and 7 percent complained about government regulations.

A 1989 study by the AMA found that physicians' office staffs spent an average of 46.7 hours per month processing Medicare claims and 32.6 hours per month processing Blue Cross/Blue Shield claims.[49] Additional time is required for them to complete forms for other commercial insurers. Physicians estimated that it took nearly one hour of staff time for each claim submitted to Medicare or Blue Cross/Blue Shield. In addition, the typical physician personally must spend 4.6 hours per month on administrative work related to Medicare claims and 2.4 hours per month on similar work related to Blue Cross/Blue Shield claims. Nearly 14 percent of the 3,000

[48]Kenneth H. Bacon, "Doctors Chafe at Changes in Medicare, Expecting More Paper Work, Less Money," *Wall Street Journal*, August 22, 1990.

[49]American Medical Association, *Socioeconomic Monitoring System Report* 3, no. 2 (1989).

physicians who participated in the study reported that they had resorted to using outside billing services to file claims or help meet reporting requirements and regulations.

Dr. Gordon Leitch, an eye surgeon in Tigard, Oregon, commented in an interview that "increased paperwork due to insurance and HMOs has intruded upon my and my staff's time available to provide health care. HMOs and other third-party payment have an effect on raising health care costs due to the extra layer of bureaucracy they generate."[50] Sheila Nabil, a registered nurse working with family practitioners in Virginia, remarked that nurses are seeing an increased amount of paperwork, particularly with HMOs, and that it affects the amount of time they can spend with patients.[51]

Delaware orthopedist Stephen Hershey complained that he must employ several staff members who do nothing but paperwork for insurance.[52] And Pennsylvania family practitioner Richard Bruehlman reported that

> paperwork required by third-party payers has forced our group to computerize business and demographic data, at a cost of close to $100,000! We have three full-time employees who do nothing but handle business matters; one of these employees works solely on HMO issues. I should add that insurance considerations enter conversations that I have with patients, decreasing the amount of time spent on history taking, exams, and patient education.[53]

Perhaps Paul Glanville, the Arizona family practitioner mentioned in the introduction, said it best by giving a short history of the 20th-century physician:

> Doc had to hire a secretary because his office isn't in the home anymore; he can't make house calls because it isn't cost effective; and he has to add a back office assistant to be more efficient because he has to make more money to pay the increased overhead of an office outside the home and the secretary. The insurance is getting more complicated, and he has to accept insurance, so it takes more paperwork and time so he has to add a part-time assistant for just that.

[50]From correspondence with the author.
[51]From interview with the author.
[52]From correspondence with the author.
[53]From correspondence with the author.

He has to add a small computer to keep track of all the insurance billing; then the HMO/PPOs come in and take a discount, and the paperwork mounts up and becomes so complicated that he needs a bigger computer and fancy software to keep track of it all; but he needs another assistant who is computer literate, so he has to see more patients to pay for this. But the HMO takes such a large discount that it takes twice as many patients to pay for the increase so he needs another back office assistant; but with the increase in patients he needs a larger office with more exam rooms, and his old loan was almost paid off at the low interest rate, but now he has a larger loan with much higher interest and he needs to see more patients and hire more people. . . . And the barriers go up, separating the doctor from those in need.[54]

The Deteriorating Doctor-Patient Relationship

Physicians are concerned about the decline in the doctor-patient relationship that has occurred over the past few decades. They complain that the increase in bureaucracy and paperwork associated with both government programs and insurance companies has cut into the time they have to spend with patients (a concern also registered by nursing staffs). Because HMOs limit their reimbursements on physician charges, doctors must see increased numbers of patients to turn a profit or, in some cases, to break even. Caps on Medicare charges have the same result, and doctors are increasingly frustrated with such intrusions on their time.

Physicians and nursing staffs also are concerned that the inexpensive copayments[55] required by HMOs for office visits encourage overutilization of medical care. Sheila Nabil, a nurse formerly in the military, has noted that both in the military and in private practice she has seen patients who make unnecessary visits to the doctor for problems that are self-treatable or that would eventually disappear without treatment.[56] She believes that the low copayments normally associated with HMOs, and the free care in the military, encourage this overuse of the health care system. Dr.

[54]From correspondence with the author.

[55]A copayment is the amount that the patient is required to pay at the time services are rendered, usually a nominal amount ($5 or $10).

[56]From interview with the author.

Michael Filak, a family practitioner in Virginia, stated that he frequently sees overuse of medical care services that he attributes to low copayments.[57]

Some physicians express concern that they have difficulty developing long-term relationships with their patients, primarily because patients switch HMOs and insurance plans with increasing frequency. Most people receive their health insurance coverage through their employer, and when they change jobs or their employer discontinues using a particular insurance company, they must switch plans. Often, when a patient changes insurance coverage, his or her current physician does not accept the new plan and the patient must find a new physician.

Physicians say that losing patients to insurance and job changes is a significant problem in their practices. Dr. Richard Bruehlman, for example, added that "the lack of a long-term relationship fragments the continuity of care of a patient, which I feel is arguably the single most important aspect of quality medical care. Continuity of care also has been demonstrated to decrease costs."[58] Dr. Cheryl Rosenblatt, an allergist practicing in Maryland and Virginia, agreed, saying that "changing HMOs raises costs on the entire system—for example, if a new patient comes to me because of an insurance change, many times I have to retest for allergies even though they may have just had testing, because the new HMO requires it."[59]

Perhaps one of the biggest concerns for physicians is the change many see in how patients relate to their doctors. Some physicians feel, possibly because of the increased use of technology and large malpractice awards, that patient expectations for care are too high, that they expect the doctor to be able to fix anything. According to Rosenblatt, "Patients have unrealistic expectations. They expect miracles out of doctors. Malpractice intrudes the most on the doctor-patient relationship. I don't like looking at patients as adversaries."[60]

Some doctors comment that patients are less trusting and more demanding of physicians. Others complain that HMOs and insurance companies pit doctor against patient by denying access to

[57]From interview with the author.

[58]From correspondence with the author.

[59]From interview with the author.

[60]From interview with the author.

specialists and by second-guessing decisions regarding treatment. However, Tennessee orthopedic surgeon Paul Parsons remarked that for him the situation was different:

> Now the doctor and the patient have a new adversary besides disease that they must join together against to defeat—that is the government and the third-party payer that would deny care. I have made as many longtime friends in private practice by helping them combat the system as I have by curing their physical maladies.[61]

Second-Guessing the Physician

Many physicians are fed up with bureaucracy, interference with their practice of medicine, and harassment of both themselves and their staffs by government and private insurance companies. Denials of payment, demands to justify clinical judgments, and requirements for prior approval undermine professional decisionmaking and physician-patient relationships. Physicians could better use the time and money they spend responding to insurance carriers' and quality review organizations' demands for documentation and justification to improve patient care and enhance their medical knowledge and skill.

One of the main targets of their frustration is the so-called utilization review, a term used to cover the numerous programs, such as screenings of hospital admissions and medical tests, that insurers, employers, and other third-party payers adopted in the 1980s to cut health costs. "One physician may have to deal with 10 to 20 different review organizations a day, each of which has unique criteria" for evaluating medical claims, said John T. Kelly, director of the AMA's office of quality assurance.[62] Such numerous interactions eat into physician and staff time and are typically confusing and exasperating. As John Koch, the Johns Hopkins otolaryngologist said, "The need for approval for individual items of diagnostic work-up and therapy is unwieldy."[63]

Physicians are also tired of being second-guessed on medical treatment decisions by nonmedical personnel, which can frequently

[61]From correspondence with the author.

[62]Quoted in Glenn Ruffenach, "Doctors, Review Firms Try to See Eye to Eye" *Wall Street Journal*, March 3, 1990.

[63]From correspondence with the author.

result in denials of claims for treatment by either the government or insurance companies. Such denials have angered both doctors and patients and have even resulted in some lawsuits filed by both physicians and patients against insurance companies. According to Tennessee surgeon Paul Parsons:

> Increasingly, HMOs and private insurance carriers are dictating medical care in this country based solely on financial concerns. Physicians are faced with two choices in diagnosing and treating their patients. The first choice is to function independently, ordering such tests and treatments as are deemed necessary and paying no heed to the objections raised by the HMOs. The second choice is to alter their medical care and judgment to comply with the ever-changing rules and regulations of the HMOs and insurance carriers. These third-party payers do indeed influence and change the care delivered at the grass-roots level.[64]

Doctors and patients alike are concerned that second-guessing by nonmedical personnel can inhibit or lessen the quality and effectiveness of medical treatment. Many accuse health insurance companies and government programs of being more concerned about the bottom line and cutting costs than about the quality of care received by patients.

Dr. Michael Mobley, a psychiatrist practicing in Georgia, complained of harassment in dealing with the Medicare program:

> In my own psychiatric practice, which is about 50 percent geriatric, I have been "battling" with insurers to process clean claims correctly. . . . My experience has been one of cost containment through harassment. If my office manager was not prone to detail, legitimate reimbursement would have been lost to processing errors. Not unlike my colleagues, I am demoralized by the way Medicare is relating to me. The added stress from the current Medicare system in Georgia has me in active review of my commitment to geriatric psychiatry.[65]

The Malpractice Nightmare

Most physicians have something to say about the increase in malpractice suits and the exorbitant cost of liability insurance.

[64]Paul Parsons, letter to the editor, *Wall Street Journal*, March 14, 1990.
[65]Michael Mobley, letter to the editor, *Wall Street Journal*, February 2, 1990.

According to the AMA opinion surveys, 61 percent of the physicians interviewed said they were concerned about the possibility of a medical malpractice lawsuit in the next year. One of the fastest growing components of practice costs for physicians has been professional liability insurance. Average premiums for self-employed physicians have increased at an average annual rate of 21.9 percent, rising from $5,800 in 1982 to $12,800 in 1986.[66] Average liability insurance premiums in obstetrics and gynecology increased from $10,800 to $29,300 during the same period. The rise in premiums has been attributed to the increased incidence of malpractice claims and rising amounts of jury awards.[67]

Professional liability claims rose from 3.2 claims per 100 physicians before 1981 to 9.2 claims per 100 physicians in 1986, and more than one-third of all physicians had been sued at least once in their careers as of 1986.[68] Initial jury awards for both economic and noneconomic damages averaged $1,760,632 in 1987; the median award was $825,000.[69] As recently as 1980, awards averaged $404,726, and the median was $150,000.[70]

Increases in professional liability premiums have consumed a growing share of physicians' practice revenues. Rising premiums, liability claims, and awards to patients are all contributors to the rise in health care costs for everyone. Many physicians are also concerned about the effects of rising insurance costs on the quality of care. According to Dr. David Sundwall, vice president and medical director of the American Healthcare Systems Institute, "The fear of suits has driven more than half the family physicians out of obstetrics, and an increasing number of specialists in obstetrics and gynecology have chosen to limit their practice to female and reproductive surgery, and have stopped delivering babies."[71] He went on to say that that fear is why some parts of the United

[66]Center for Health Policy Research, *Socioeconomic Characteristics of Medical Practice, 1987* (Chicago, 1987).

[67]Ibid.

[68]Ibid.

[69]E. M. Solon, "Current Award Trends," in *Socio-Economic Factbook for Surgery, 1989* (Chicago: American College of Surgeons, 1989).

[70]Ibid.

[71]David Sundwall, letter to the editor, *Wall Street Journal*, November 30, 1990.

States lack such services and that their absence contributes to infant mortality problems.

Problems with Medicare

"I no longer can tolerate the limits imposed by the Medicare bureaucracy on clinical practice, patient care, and accounts receivable. Therefore, I have stopped accepting Medicare patients in my office practice," declared Dr. Edward Sodaro.[72] The Medicare program is a source of frustration and headaches; some doctors limit the number of Medicare patients they take or refuse to take them at all. Doctors complain that the program continually expands its bureaucracy and adds more regulatory requirements to their practices.

In September 1990 the Medicare program required doctors and suppliers of medical equipment to file all Medicare insurance claims for their patients at no charge, thereby adding to the mountains of paperwork under which most doctors' offices were already buried. Physicians are concerned that this requirement has added increased administrative costs to their practices. "Not only has Medicare intruded upon the patient's freedom to choose," commented Dr. Martha Stearn, an internist in Wyoming, "it has cut into the time the physician has to care for the patient. I spend far too much time filling out forms for Medicare, having to justify why I ordered home oxygen, a wheelchair, a hospital bed at home."[73] In a 1990 survey by the Association of American Physicians and Surgeons, 33 percent of the physicians responding said that the fact that doctors must now submit all claims is cause for future restrictions on accepting Medicare patients.[74]

Another change, which became effective January 1, 1991, places uniform new limits on what physicians can charge Medicare

---

[72]Edward R. Sodaro, M.D., "HCFA Policy Limits Freedom of Choice for Senior Citizens," *Private Practice*, November 1989 p. 42–43.

[73]Martha Stearn, "Medicare: Diagnosis Grim, Prognosis Grimmer," *Wall Street Journal*, June 4, 1991.

[74]*AAPS News* 46, no. 5 (May 1990) p. 1; hereinafter, the AAPS survey. Questionnaires were sent to physicians in active practice of adult patient-care specialties: 968 in Pima County, Arizona; 1,145 in Hamilton and Lucas counties, Ohio; 912 in Jefferson County, Kentucky; and 240 in De Kalb County, Georgia. There were 438 responses, covering six specialties: primary care, surgery, psychiatry, neurology, internal medicine, and dermatology.

patients. When doctors deal with Medicare patients, they can choose between two basic billing procedures. They can accept the patient on assignment, which means that they can charge the patient only what Medicare allows for each procedure, send their bill to the insurance company that handles Medicare claims in their area, and receive reimbursement. About 80 percent of Medicare's claims are submitted on assignment.

Doctors using the second method, called balance billing, charge more than the Medicare reimbursement rate, which means that the patient must pay the difference between what Medicare pays and the higher amount the doctor charges. In 1991 balance billing charges paid by patients and insurers totaled $1.9 billion.[75] On January 1, 1992, the maximum doctors could charge under balance billing was limited to 125 percent of the Medicare reimbursement rate. That cap will fall to 115 percent by 1993.

In reality this arrangement amounts to a setting of prices not by the market but by the government. Doctors who may want to charge a specific additional amount for their services are forbidden to do so, and patients who may feel it is worth paying the additional amount to be treated by the physician of their choice are not allowed to do so. A recent case epitomizes this kind of conflict. In June 1989 the U.S. Supreme Court let stand a District of Columbia Court of Appeals decision (*New York Ophthalmology Society* v. *Bowen*) that prevented a Medicare beneficiary from using his own money to pay for an allegedly superfluous service—in this case the attendance of an assistant eye surgeon during a cataract extraction.[76] When eye surgeons had been found by the Office of the Inspector General to get along without an assistant in some areas of the country, Congress had passed a law declaring the practice to be unnecessary everywhere else. An "unnecessary" service could not be a covered benefit of Medicare. The Court of Appeals extended this reasoning to make assisting during cataract surgery virtually illegal, at least for an operation on anyone over the age of 65. Although it isn't illegal for a surgeon to assist in cataract surgery, it is illegal to have anyone pay for it.

---

[75]From correspondence with the Health Care Financing Administration.

[76]Philip R. Alper, "Doctor-Patient Relationship Takes Turn for the Worse: Inside the Medicare Dictatorship," *Wall Street Journal*, January 18, 1990.

The economic result of such a regulation is that some doctors will find that they must reduce or eliminate completely the number of Medicare patients they see. The results of the AAPS survey show that some 15 percent of the physicians responding were already restricting the number of Medicare appointments they accepted. A ban on balance billing would result in up to 45 percent of the doctors surveyed decreasing the number of Medicare patients they accept for treatment.

Inadequate reimbursement for services is a complaint of many physicians who accept Medicare patients. Some physicians in the AAPS survey commented that they had quit practicing, had stopped accepting Medicare patients, or had reduced services to Medicare patients because they were unable to earn enough to cover their overhead. William Anderson, a California neurologist, had himself decertified as a Medicare provider when he found that the maximum amount he could charge under Medicare's fee-limitation rules was lower than his overhead for his most frequent services.[77] In a confusing series of letters, Region IX of the Department of Health and Human Services concluded that even though Medicare would have no further financial liability for Anderson's services, he would still have to abide by its fee limitations and all other rules whenever he treated a Medicare patient. Anderson worried that statutory penalties of up to $2,000 for every single "overcharge" might be assessed against him. He now asks Medicare patients to pay an amount equal to his normal fee to a major charity rather than to him. At the same time, he limits his care to a maximum of one Medicare patient per day.

Internist Martha Stearn, in private practice in Jackson, Wyoming, has related her own experience:

> Sylvia comes in with a heart arrhythmia. I begin to inform her that she can be treated as an outpatient. Then I remember Medicare (which will only pay for one visit per week, and the treatment would require several). So I tell Sylvia she will have to be admitted to the hospital.
>
> She protests. She doesn't feel sick enough to be hospitalized. And her son and his family are visiting. She hasn't seen them in a year. I tell her that Medicare will not pay for more than one visit per week, and she will have to see me

[77]Ibid.

more often than that. Sylvia wants to pay me from her own pocket, but I am obligated to tell her that Medicare will not allow her that choice.

She gets confused and angry. Medicare, which she once welcomed as her guardian, keeps her from getting the medical care she wants. She resents its interference.

Seeing her terrible frustration, I reconsider. We strike a deal that even Medicare cannot undermine; she will be treated as an outpatient and she will bring me her best garden tomatoes in the fall. Medicare will pay for less than half of her visits, but I will take care of her on my terms. And our tomato deal will save the taxpayer thousands of dollars.[78]

Many doctors in the AAPS survey said that they would like to retire or restrict their practices but could not afford to do so. Overall, they reported that receipts from treating Medicare patients averaged 60 percent of their normal fee charged. According to the survey, any additional cuts in reimbursement amounts would result in 47 percent of the respondents further restricting their acceptance of Medicare patients. Medicare patients in some areas of the country may already be having difficulty finding a doctor. More restrictions and costs imposed on physicians by the government may cause that difficulty to increase as more and more doctors discontinue treating or refuse to accept new Medicare patients.

Physicians who participate in the Medicare program increasingly fear being falsely accused of fraud. Any physician who accepts Medicare patients must sign a contract with the federal government. The contract states what the doctor can and cannot do in treating patients, and there are civil and criminal penalties if regulations are not followed. Problems arise because doctors often do not have the time to read the voluminous regulations published and because the regulations are frequently not published promptly or even written.

According to Dr. Carol Brown, a psychiatrist practicing in Hawaii, the ordeal of being accused of fraud can be terrifying. Because she was a highly productive physician and submitted a large number

[78]Stearn.

of bills to Medicare, she was targeted for a fraud investigation.[79] She was accused of mishandling patient care, her office was searched, and both her Medicare and private-pay-patient medical records were seized (the government ignored the facts that patient records are confidential and that the private-pay records had no bearing on the investigation). She said that her reputation as a physician has suffered irreparable damage.

Taking Early Retirement

Canada, which has operated under a system of nationalized health care for several years now, continually experiences the problem of physicians changing professions, moving to the United States, or taking early retirement. However, the problem of physicians leaving their field is not restricted to Canada. Increasingly, physicians' frustration with bureaucratic hassles, too much paperwork, malpractice worries, and a whole host of other irritations is resulting in the withdrawal of U.S. physicians from the practice of medicine. Seventy percent of the physicians in the AAPS survey said that they were considering early retirement from their chosen profession. The proportion was somewhat lower (57 percent), but still significant, for those in practice five or fewer years.

Some physicians would quit medicine if the United States adopted a national health care system like that found in Canada. A physician in California remarked that he felt confident that the United States would quickly abandon a Canadian-type system and that he would return to practice as soon as it was revoked. Another physician, who would continue to practice, said he would not participate in the nationalized system but would barter goods for medical care if he had to in order to remain in private practice.

Things are so bad that some physicians say they would recommend that their children not become physicians.[80] One remarked

---

[79]This account is excerpted from a lecture given by Dr. Carol Brown at the annual meeting of the Association of American Physicians and Surgeons, Scottsdale, Arizona, September 1990. See *AAPS News* 46, no. 11 (November 1990): 1.

[80]In the 1990 AMA opinion surveys, 58 percent of physicians asked said they would recommend medicine as a career choice to a high school or college student, and 38 percent said they would not. Of those saying they would not, 42 percent cited "outside interference" and "regulation" as the main reasons. In the 1991 *Washingtonian* survey, 38 percent of physicians interviewed said they would not encourage a student to go into medicine, stating that the rewards are not worth the emotional and physical costs.

that he told his son that to become a physician today meant "becoming a slave to non-medical bosses, politicians, and bureaucrats."[81] His son went into the medical profession anyway.

Tennessee surgeon Paul Parsons related what he would tell his teenage son or daughter:

> Would I recommend you practice medicine? What does that mean? First of all, it means hard work and top grades in high school. This continues for four years of college. No time for parties, football games, dances, or dating. Assuming you've worked hard enough to get in, medical school is four years of trying to learn the basics of all fields of medicine. This is nearly impossible and requires continuous study. Hardly time for a family.
>
> We haven't even talked about expense yet. You finish medical school, you're twenty-six years old, have four to eight years of training left before you can charge your first patient, and you're fifty to one hundred thousand dollars in debt! Did I mention the exposure to hepatitis and AIDS?
>
> Now, let's assume you choose orthopedics. That means five additional years of residency, working one hundred hours a week for less than minimum wage. Did I mention the government no longer allows deferment of student loans during residency?
>
> Finally, at age thirty-one, you start your practice, see your first patient who needs an operation, and you're told over the phone by a high school dropout working for an insurance company that you can't do the operation! What would I tell you to do? Put the same time, energy, and effort into a small business and retire at age thirty-one![82]

And Wyoming internist Martha Stearn has warned that "as the government's hold on the physician's and the patient's autonomy tightens, more and more doctors are finding ways to opt out. The security of a salary. A career change. A disappointing early retirement. The physician can escape. The patient cannot. And ultimately it is the patient who suffers."[83]

[81]Dr. John Toth, in correspondence with the author.
[82]From correspondence with the author.
[83]Stearn.

The Hospitals

Hospitals find themselves increasingly squeezed by regulation, the cost of uncompensated care, and pressure from Medicare and insurance companies.

The Cost of Regulation

"Hospitals usually operate on the margin," said Steven Brown, administrator of Fair Oaks Hospital in Fairfax, Virginia, "and one piece of legislation could kill you."[84] On this day he was speaking about a recent law passed by the Virginia state legislature requiring that all infectious waste be boxed as well as bagged. Brown was concerned about the increased costs to the hospital of complying with the additional boxing requirement.

The ever-increasing costs of health care are affecting the nation's hospitals, and the explosion of regulations from and bureaucracy in both government and insurance companies is pushing the operating margin of most hospitals, and the patience of their employees, to the breaking point. Consider, for example, the case of Sequoia Hospital, a 430-bed, not-for-profit general hospital in San Francisco. According to Dr. Sidney Marchasin, vice president of the board of directors of the hospital: "The groans you hear coming from your local hospital are not all emanating from patients. They're the protests of nurses, hospital personnel and physicians who are forced to live with a hodgepodge of expensive, contradictory and confusing bureaucratic regulations."[85]

Marchasin contended that the federal government is responsible for many of the costs that confound the health care industry, because it is the legislators and bureaucrats who document deficiencies in the system and then invoke numerous rules, regulations, and paperwork. He calculated that the price tag for dealing with various regulatory bodies and paperwork at Sequoia is approximately $7.8 million annually.[86]

Although the number of patients at Sequoia is the same as it was in 1966, the staff is about 75 percent larger than it was then. To comply with the regulations and government directives requires a

[84]From interview with the author.

[85]Sidney Marchasin, "One Hospital Tells the Cost of Regulation," *Wall Street Journal*, June 26, 1990.

[86]Ibid.

staff of 140 full-time employees. Marchasin did not include in that figure the number of physician hours devoted to helping the hospital comply with mandated government audits and utilization review programs. Marchasin went on to say that

> the Federal Peer Review Act mandates that all hospital work paid for by the government be reviewed by an independent agency under contract to the Health Care Financing Administration. Providing duplicate hospital records, lab reports, X-ray data and billing information to outside peer review agencies is an enormous task requiring 20 additional staffers. As for Medicare funds, to get those the hospital must undergo a third audit, by the Joint Commission on Accreditation of Health Care Organizations.[87]

Every auditing agency issues further regulations, generating more paperwork that must be filled out by nurses, hospital pharmacists, record-room personnel, and physicians. To lighten the paperwork load, Sequoia Hospital added four people to the medical staff office and three data processors.

"If Sequoia's experience is typical," wrote Marchasin, "and there's no reason to suspect it is not—health-care regulatory costs nationwide measure in the billions of dollars. Excessive regulatory activity has not only failed to produce a health-care system to carry us into the next century; it has weakened what we already have."[88]

Marchasin then suggested a solution, perhaps born out of regulatory frustration:

> The best way to start solving the health-care cost crisis is to suggest that many of the government's regulators resign en masse, and then accept these resignations so fast they don't even have time to hit the table. The patients would not lose much of value. And I would surmise that people would be much happier knowing their taxes were being spent on older people's medical needs rather than on a massive government bureaucracy.[89]

[87]Ibid.
[88]Ibid.
[89]Ibid.

Uncompensated Care

Traditionally, many doctors and hospitals have given free or below-cost treatment to the indigent and have covered the cost by charging more to patients who are able to pay. Similarly, indigent patients not eligible for government programs have been subsidized in effect by padded bills for patients covered by Medicaid. But the adoption of cost-control efforts, such as prospective payment and capitation, by Medicare and by state Medicaid programs, together with employers' exerting greater pressure on hospitals to limit their charges to private group-insured patients, have increased the indigent-care problem. Closer scrutiny by insurers and businesses of the hospital bills of their private patients prevents hospitals from charging more to privately insured patients to finance indigent care. Hospitals are faced with absorbing the cost of treating these patients or dumping them (discharging them early or sending them to another hospital).

Nationally, hospitals provided more than $11.5 billion in uncompensated care in 1990, up from $3.9 billion in 1980.[90] Hospitals also absorbed the cost of more than $6 billion in charity care in 1990.[91] For Steven Brown, administrator at Fair Oaks Hospital, uncompensated care is a "significant problem," totaling $2 million to $3 million per year.[92] In Washington, D.C., for example, unpaid hospital bills run over $100 million a year.[93]

Problems with Reimbursement from Insurance Companies

In addition to their decreased ability to shift costs because of the regulatory limits imposed by government, hospitals are finding that many of their charges are being challenged by private companies and insurance groups. Springing up across the country are companies that review the cost of drugs and procedures on hospital bills and recommend that their clients—mostly insurance firms—refuse to make payment on part of the tab. Some of these cases have resulted in lawsuits filed by hospitals, which claim that they have been unfairly denied payment.

[90]American Hospital Association, *Annual Survey of Hospitals*, 1980–1989.

[91]Data from the American Hospital Association.

[92]From interview with the author.

[93]"Crisis of the Emergency Rooms" (editorial), *Washington Post*, September 10, 1989.

Michael D. Stephens, president and chief executive of Hoag Memorial Presbyterian Hospital in Newport Beach, California, has explained that such companies assume that hospitals price their services like a store.[94] However, besides paying part of the hospital's overhead for equipment, nursing, and administration, each patient must share the burden of providing free treatment to needy people, said Stephens. Thus, when a hospital charges $6 for an aspirin, it is apportioning total costs to help cover the price of uncompensated care.

The Construction Dilemma

The construction of hospitals in the United States over the past several decades has been on a virtual merry-go-round. Although many people in Congress and the government are now saying that we have too many hospitals that employ too much high technology and provide excess hospital beds, the very same government has done much to encourage hospital construction over the years. The cost of completed hospital construction projects totaled $16.3 billion in 1989, up 19 percent from 1988 ($13.7 billion), according to a survey by *Modern Healthcare*.[95] Federal subsidies accounted for approximately $5.8 billion of the cost.[96]

The Hospital Survey and Construction Act of 1946 (Hill-Burton Act), before its expiration in 1978, provided $4.4 billion in federal money as leverage to encourage state and local governments to contribute an additional $9.1 billion toward hospital construction, resulting in the creation of 500,000 beds. The recent building boom is very much a product of the enactment of Medicare for the elderly and Medicaid for the poor nearly 25 years ago. The new coverage has provided a steady flow of federal funds to hospitals. In addition, Medicare agreed to reimburse hospitals for reasonable capital costs incurred to provide care for the elderly. With guaranteed federal funding, hospitals could easily borrow money.

Before Medicare, hospitals raised most of their money from charitable contributions. Because the sources of capital in the past were

[94]Rhonda L. Rundle, "Hospital Groups Try to Pull Off Cost Watchdogs," *Wall Street Journal*, August 16, 1989.

[95]"Modern Healthcare, 1990 Construction and Architects Survey," *Modern Healthcare*, February 19, 1990.

[96]Ibid.

individual contributors, a hospital was careful in developing building plans, erecting only as much physical plant as appeared necessary at the time. The switch to public financing made it easier to finance expansion and led to overcapitalization in the industry.

After encouraging hospital construction for decades, the government now is attempting to reverse the steamroller it set in motion. One example is legislation introduced by Reps. Pete Stark (D-Calif.) and Brian Donnelly (D-Mass.) that would reduce excess bed capacity by penalizing hospitals that have low occupancy rates by reducing their Medicare capital reimbursements—just the opposite of what the government has been doing. Although not all hospitals responded to the government stimuli, the government's decision to call a halt is throwing many hospitals into a crunch.

Problems with Medicare/Medicaid Reimbursement

Medicare's system of diagnostic related groups (DRGs) for reimbursing hospitals causes them to receive less than what is necessary to cover their operating expenses.[97] As health care costs continue to rise year after year, it becomes increasingly difficult for most hospitals to make ends meet. "Hospitals will be faced with two choices," said Steven Brown of Fair Oaks Hospital. "Either they will not be able to afford to see as many elderly Medicare patients, or a two-tiered system will develop within the hospital where people who can pay full-price will get better care."[98]

Hospitals in various states are having trouble obtaining reimbursement from their state Medicaid programs. The Massachusetts Hospital Association has sued the governor and other state health officials for not forking over payments for Medicaid bills. The Michigan Hospital Association has sued that state for the same reason. Three Colorado hospitals won a suit against Colorado for unpaid Medicaid bills. As Irene Frazier of the American Hospital Association has explained, "In most states the amount of reimbursement is below costs . . . [and because most state governments are under budgetary pressures,] one place they're inclined to look is Medicaid reimbursement."[99]

---

[97] A fixed schedule of fees is established by Medicare to pay hospitals for the treatment of each of 475 DRGs of illnesses. If the actual cost to the hospital is less than the DRG fee, the hospital keeps the difference; if more, it absorbs the loss.

[98] From interview with the author.

[99] "Grabbing Medicaid's Money" (editorial), *Wall Street Journal*, September 5, 1989.

Shortfalls resulting from lower reimbursements force hospitals to try to shift costs. The Massachusetts lawsuit alleges that slow payments have resulted in a $350 million backlog of payments to hospitals. "The holdup in payments is being used to balance the state budget," said William T. McGrail, vice president and general counsel of the Massachusetts Hospital Association. "They're holding up on hospital payments because they don't have the cash."[100] But the backlog in payments has caused a number of hospitals to have difficulty in staffing and in providing adequate care.

According to the American Hospital Association, Medicaid payments consistently lag behind costs, and the gap has been widening in recent years.[101] Between 1980 and 1985, Medicaid paid about 90 percent of the cost of care for its beneficiaries (about three-quarters of hospital charges for those patients). By 1989 payments covered only 78 percent of costs (about 55 percent of hospital charges). In 1980 hospital losses from Medicaid underpayments were $700 million; by 1989 those losses had risen to $4.3 billion.

In 1984, 39.1 percent of hospitals were receiving Medicaid payments that met their costs, and therefore they had no Medicaid shortfall. By 1989 payments were covering costs in only 12.7 percent of hospitals. In other words, by 1989 almost 9 of every 10 hospitals were losing money caring for Medicaid patients.

The AHA's analysis shows that most of the recent growth in the unreimbursed costs hospitals incur by caring for the poor has been caused by rising Medicaid losses rather than by increased losses from patients with no payment source. In 1989 Medicaid patients accounted for only 11 percent of total hospital expenses but a third of hospital losses attributable to caring for the poor. With the continued growth in Medicaid losses, hospitals are likely to find it more and more difficult to provide care for patients with no insurance at all.

Managed-Care Programs

The problems with managed-care program patients, such as those who belong to HMOs, are similar to the difficulties encountered with Medicare and Medicaid. Managed-care programs bring

[100]Ibid.

[101]The data presented in this paragraph and the following two paragraphs are from American Hospital Association, *Annual Survey of Hospitals*, 1980–1989; and American Hospital Association, "Medicaid Underpayments and Hospital Care for the Poor: A Fact Sheet" (January 1991).

patients to the hospitals, which generates business, but that business is at a discount (lower reimbursement levels). Hospitals are forced to make up the difference somewhere else, usually on private-pay patients, or they must absorb the cost. The increase in the number of managed-care patients, along with those on government programs, has made it tougher for hospitals to operate in the black.

Conclusion

Most patients seem satisfied with the quality of health care as long as they are adequately insured, and most Americans are. They like their doctors, but they are concerned about rising costs and those who can't afford care or obtain insurance. According to some opinion polls, however, they apparently have "more want than wallet for the problem."[102] Most doctors are happy practicing medicine (treating patients) but are increasingly unhappy with all the bureaucratic and financial hassles. Hospitals, laboring under heavy regulation, rising costs, and declining incomes, are simply trying to stay afloat.

[102]Quote attributed to President George Bush and cited in Stevens.

3. A History of Government and Health Care

How did we weave ourselves such a tangled web? What flaws within our health care system have caused patients and medical personnel to become dissatisfied with aspects of our health care system? How *did* we get here from there?

An investigation of the evolution of the medical industry in the United States will uncover clues to the predicament in which we find ourselves. It will expose not the competitive market that most Americans assume has been operating, but stifling regulation and government control—regulations originating from interest groups such as medical organizations and insurance companies, resulting in a chaotic system for both doctors and patients. What appears to most to be a free-market operation is really an industry legislated and regulated from behind the scenes. As Ayn Rand once remarked, "The concept of *free* competition enforced by law is a grotesque contradiction in terms."[1]

The Early Years (before 1930)

The federal government's involvement in health care started long before the 20th century. In 1863, in the throes of the Civil War, Congress established the National Academy of Sciences to research and study health care issues. In 1878, the year that 4,000 citizens died in New Orleans and 5,000 died in Memphis, Tennessee, from a yellow fever epidemic, Congress passed the National Quarantine Services Act. In 1889 Congress appropriated a sum of $100,000 to aid victims of yellow fever, a figure that by 1893 had grown to the $1 million mark and expanded to include other epidemic diseases. President Theodore Roosevelt created several commissions on health care and was instrumental in the passage of several pieces

[1]Ayn Rand, "Antitrust: The Rule of Unreason," *Objectivist Newsletter* 1, no. 2 (February 1962): 5.

of legislation, such as the Pure Food and Drug Act and the Meat Inspection Act. Between 1921 and 1929 the Sheppard-Towner Act provided public health assistance to mothers and children, and many health professionals involved in that program went on to become involved with President Franklin D. Roosevelt's New Deal health programs.

The Federal Government and Health Care

Long before the federal government became involved in controlling epidemics and providing care to the indigent, the colonies were caring for their veterans.[2] In 1636 Plymouth, Massachusetts, passed a law that any soldier wounded by Indians would be taken care of for life by the colony. The Continental Congress passed legislation providing for the care of soldiers disabled in combat, although the emphasis was on pensions, not medical care.

Most post-Revolutionary War medical treatment was provided by the states or local communities. However, in 1799 President John Adams signed the Act for Relief of Sick and Disabled Seamen, which was the beginning of the U.S. Marine Service (the precursor to the U.S. Public Health Service). That act provided care for sick seamen and also made provision for the building of hospitals, the first of which was the Boston Marine Hospital, built in 1804. In an early mixing of health care and politics, the director of the Boston Marine Hospital was accused of nepotism and of setting up a monopoly on cowpox vaccine, and President James Madison was forced to fire him.

In 1811 the first medical facilities were provided for naval veterans, and in 1842 the Navy formed the Bureau of Medicine and Surgery. By 1813 the Army had established the Office of Physician and Surgeon General. In 1851 Congress authorized the first federal homes for disabled soldiers. Fifteen years later, Congress established the National Asylum (the name was later changed to "Home") for Disabled Volunteer Soldiers, which would provide care for indigent and disabled veterans.

In 1870 President Ulysses S. Grant placed the hospitals within the Marine Hospital Service under the direction of the first surgeon

---

[2]The sources for this section include the Department of Health, Education, and Welfare, *Health in America 1776–1976* (Washington: 1976); and Paul Starr, *The Social Transformation of American Medicine* (New York: Basic Books, 1982).

general, Dr. John Woodworth. In 1879 Congress passed legislation creating the National Board of Health. From 1891 to 1911 Walter Wyman was surgeon general of what came to be known as the U.S. Public Health Service. He was an advocate of federal control over state and local quarantine services and a believer in federal medical research. During his tenure, public health officers were even dispatched overseas to examine potential immigrants before they embarked on the ocean voyage to the United States. However, in spite of his predisposition to federal involvement, Wyman relentlessly opposed the creation of a federal department of health.

Following World War I, the return of 5 million veterans, many of whom needed medical assistance, exceeded the current capacity of the agencies providing benefits. Congress responded by establishing the Veterans' Bureau in 1921. And in 1929 President Herbert Hoover consolidated the Pension Bureau, the National Home for Disabled Volunteer Soldiers, and the Veterans' Bureau into what is now the Department of Veterans' Affairs.

Much of the history of the U.S. public health system is a record of struggles over the limits of its mandate.[3] By the end of the 19th century, the lines between the activities of the medical profession and the public health agencies had begun to blur. Extending the boundaries of public health to incorporate more of medicine became a natural progression, but many doctors fought this usurpation of their duties. What had begun as a government program to control epidemics gradually encroached upon doctors' domain of treating the sick. Public health services expanded to include vaccinations, school health programs, and plans for public health centers in the early 1900s.

Rumblings for the adoption of national health insurance began to be heard in the early 1900s. The Commission on Industrial Relations, created by President Woodrow Wilson in the wake of labor violence, recommended health insurance in its report. The labor committee of the House of Representatives held hearings on a resolution introduced by its sole Socialist party member to create a national social insurance commission. Organizations of public health officers and nurses endorsed the proposal. And although a national health plan was not enacted, the federal government

[3]Starr, p. 180.

continued its expansion into the health care arena with the advent of President Roosevelt's New Deal programs in the 1930s and President Lyndon Johnson's Great Society programs in the 1960s.

The Rise of Today's Physician and the Advent of the American Medical Association

During the 19th century a physician's duties consisted primarily of handholding and comforting both patient and family as the illness from which the patient was suffering took its natural course. Louis Pasteur's proof of the germ theory of disease in 1862 and the discovery of anesthesia in the mid-19th century began a revolution in the practice of medicine. As a result of Pasteur's theory, Joseph Lister introduced the use of antiseptics during operations, followed by the use of rubber gloves and surgical masks. Another key advance was the discovery of X-rays by Wilhelm Roentgen in 1898.

By the turn of the century the role of the physician was changing dramatically from that of comforter to that of actual dispenser of treatment through surgery and the prescription of more potent medicines. As medical breakthroughs continued to occur, schools were developed to teach the new techniques. Very important for American medicine was the establishment of a medical program at Johns Hopkins University by William Osler in 1888. According to author and physician Lewis Thomas, Osler and his colleagues pointed out that most of the remedies in common use were more likely to do harm than good, and that there were only a small number of genuine therapeutic drugs—and they laid out a new, highly conservative curriculum for training medical students.[4] The curriculum taught at Johns Hopkins became the model for all American medical schools. Yet, during the first decades of the 20th century, most medical students preferred to study in Germany and Austria, still considered the leading centers of medical education.

The American Medical Association was first established as a national organization in 1847. The AMA's stated goals were to raise the quality of care of patients and protect consumers from the activities of charlatans. However, beneath the surface there was a strong concern—expressed by many members—with maintaining the financial stability and superiority of the physician. Thus began

[4]Lewis Thomas, *The Youngest Science: Notes of a Medicine-Watcher* (New York: Viking Press, 1983), p. 20.

the development of a relationship between the government and the AMA that has continued to the present day, a relationship that involves government protection of the organization's stature through legislation and regulation.[5]

In the beginning, no physician was permitted to have direct membership in the AMA. Physicians were members of county medical societies, and acceptance was determined by whether or not the physician was a reputable and ethically licensed medical doctor. The medical school conferred the degree, the state determined licensure, but the county society decided who was reputable and ethical. (Only recently has the AMA permitted direct membership.)

Most physicians joined the AMA because they felt they had to in order to practice. In the early days, AMA membership was a necessity; hospital privileges, the ability to get insurance, and even the right to join the Navy were dependent on AMA membership. The AMA quickly became one of the most powerful trade associations in America, more powerful than many unions. The AMA's Council on Medical Education controlled the medical schools by increasing standards for accreditation—driving some schools out of business and discouraging new ones—and by dictating curricula.

The AMA's state medical societies nominate the physicians who serve on the state licensing boards. That practice allows the societies to determine the standards of medical practice and bar those they feel are not qualified. This arrangement has resulted in restrictions on the practices of health professionals such as nurses, physical therapists, clinical psychologists, chiropractors, and pharmacists. According to Dr. Thomas Ainsworth, a California surgeon general, "Organized medicine has clearly created a monopoly for the M.D. as the legitimate healer in American society. Legislation enacted over the years to protect the profession's position has almost [ensured] the continuation of this enviable status."[6]

The AMA argues that licensure assists consumers in distinguishing the qualified from the quack. In reality, licensure often endangers patients by making them less watchful because they assume

---

[5]For a more detailed account of the relationship between the AMA and government, see John C. Goodman, *The Regulation of Medical Care: Is the Price Too High?* (Washington: Cato Institute, 1980).

[6]Thomas H. Ainsworth, *Live or Die* (New York: Macmillan, 1983), p. 21.

41

that any licensed physician must be competent. Most state licensing laws permit the physician to perform all types of health services, even those for which he is not specifically trained. Some states do not require any continuing education, so once a doctor is licensed, he or she may or may not stay abreast of the latest medical knowledge and information.[7] Typically, once a physician receives his or her medical license, it is almost never revoked, unless the physician is convicted of breaking the law.

Licensing laws raise the price of entry, thereby benefiting current practitioners. Such laws provide a control on the supply of physicians, and they are aggressively supported by the medical societies.

Licensing laws in most states restrict the ability of physicians to advertise prices for health services. Advertising is considered unprofessional when engaged in by a single physician. Advertisements that promote the medical community in general, however, are acceptable. The restriction on advertising is supported by medical societies because it constrains the ability of doctors to compete in the area of prices, again protecting doctors' incomes. Physicians engaging in price competition have been severely punished, either by expulsion from the medical society or even by license suspension or revocation.

According to a study of the early development of licensing laws in the United States (1875–1900), the goals of the AMA in supporting licensing appeared to be to (1) establish medical licensing laws that would restrict entry into the profession and thus secure a more stable financial climate for physicians than had existed under uninhibited competition; (2) destroy the for-profit medical schools and replace them with a few nonprofit institutions that would provide extensive, thorough training in medicine over a longer required period of study to a smaller and more select student body at a higher cost; and (3) eliminate other medical sects, such as homeopaths and chiropractors, who were generally viewed as unwelcome competitive forces within the profession.[8]

The Flexner Report of 1910 further restricted entry into the medical profession. Abraham Flexner, the former owner of a Kentucky

[7]Edward H. Forgotson, Ruth Roemer, and Roger Newman, "Licensure of Physicians," *Washington University Law Quarterly* 1967 (1967): 269.

[8]Ronald Hamowy, "The Early Development of Medical Licensing Laws in the United States, 1875–1900," *Journal of Libertarian Studies* 3, no. 1 (1979): 75.

preparatory school and not a physician, was commissioned by the Carnegie Foundation to write a study of American medical education. The brother of Dr. Simon Flexner, a physician and head of the Rockefeller Institute for Medical Research, Abraham Flexner worked closely with the AMA in preparing his analysis, and the report was virtually a repetition of a 1906 evaluation of medical schools by the AMA's Council on Medical Education. The recommendations in the report were embraced by every state in the nation, and soon every school and hospital was subjected to licensing by the state, which turned the power to appoint licensing boards over to the state AMA. Legislators were convinced by the Flexner Report that only graduates of first-class medical schools ought to be licensed, and the classification of schools was delegated to the AMA. In time, every state established standards of acceptability for licensing doctors.

Through the Flexner Report the AMA was able to use government to cartelize the medical profession and raise medical and hospital prices and doctors' incomes. Ultimately, medical schools that failed to meet the high educational standards established by the AMA were closed. The AMA was successful in reducing the number of medical schools in the United States from 131 in 1910 to 85 in 1920, to 76 in 1930, and to 69 in 1944.[9]

The Flexner Report had a profound effect on future physicians from minority groups.[10] In 1910 there were seven medical schools that specialized in training black physicians, and between 1900 and 1920 the percentage of black physicians increased sharply—from 1.3 percent to 2 percent. However, between 1910 and 1944 the number of black medical schools fell from seven to two, and the proportion of black physicians among all physicians leveled off at its 1910 peak. The number of women in medical schools did not return to pre-Flexner levels until after 1940. And in the 1930s,

[9]Reuben A. Kessel, "Price Discrimination in Medicine," *Journal of Law and Economics* 1 (October 1958): 28.

[10]The data in the text are found in Goodman, pp. 30–31. For additional information on minority physicians, see Reuben A. Kessel, "The AMA and the Supply of Physicians," *Law and Contemporary Problems* (Spring 1970): 269; Richard H. Shryock, "Women in American Medicine," *Journal of the American Medical Women's Association* 5 (1950): 377; and Jacob A. Goldberg, "Jews in the Medical Profession—A National Survey," *Jewish Social Studies* 1 (1939): 332.

WHAT HAS GOVERNMENT DONE TO OUR HEALTH CARE?

because it was difficult for Jews to be admitted to U.S. medical schools, 90 percent of Americans studying medicine abroad were Jewish.

During the Great Depression the AMA exercised its power over medical schools to encourage a reduction in the number of students. As the incomes of physicians began to fall, the AMA responded with a report that exposed a purported oversupply of doctors.[11] Soon after, the AMA's Council on Medical Education surveyed 89 schools and found that many had more students than they supposedly could adequately train. The AMA exerted pressure on these schools, and acceptances to medical school declined 17.9 percent between 1933 and 1939.[12] Reuben Kessel remarked on the effects of such control:

> The delegation by the state legislature to the AMA of the power to regulate the medical industry in the public interest is on a par with giving the American Iron and Steel Institute the power to determine the output of steel. It is this power that has been given to the AMA that is the cornerstone of the monopoly power that has been imputed by economists to organized medicine.[13]

The Growth of Hospitals and the Birth of Health Insurance

Until the 20th century, hospitals were places where people went to die, not to receive treatment. They were also dangerous places to be if one was sick. An 1870 English study concluded that the death rate from surgery was higher in the hospital than in the home.[14] With the advent of antiseptics and aseptic practices in the latter part of the 19th century, hospitals greatly improved their sanitary conditions and more people went home alive after surgery. Americans began to view hospitals not as places to die but as facilities for meeting the health needs of the public.

[11]*Final Report of the Commission on Medical Education* (New York, 1932), vol. 13, p. 100.

[12]Elton Rayack, "Restrictive Practices of Organized Medicine," *Antitrust Bulletin* 13 (Summer 1968): 675.

[13]Kessel, "Price Discrimination in Medicine," p. 29.

[14]Joseph A. Califano, Jr., *America's Health Care Revolution* (New York: Random House, 1986), p. 37.

44

The growth in the number of hospitals during this period was phenomenal. In 1873 there were only 178 hospitals in the United States. In just 50 years, by 1923, the number had soared to 6,830.[15] Most of the new hospitals built between 1890 and 1920 were financed by religious organizations and charities.

During this time, Europe was turning to national health care systems and social insurance to meet its health care needs. Similar plans were proposed in the United States but failed to win support owing to Congress's suspicion of socialist policies and the public's belief in limited government. Before 1930 most Americans paid most of their medical expenses out of their own pocket, but as early as 1900 various employers, unions, and fraternal groups had begun to offer health insurance plans, and the "corporate doctor" began to appear in many companies.

The first organizations to appoint company doctors were railroad and mining companies. As accident rates rose in industry, steel makers and other manufacturers adopted the practice too. The role of the company doctor was confined mainly to the surgical repair of victims of industrial accidents. By the early 1900s industrial doctors had begun to conduct periodic as well as preemployment health examinations. Employers saw a practical side to using medical services for recruiting and selecting workers, maintaining their capacity and motivation to work, keeping down liability and insurance costs, and gaining goodwill from their employees and the public.

By the 1920s organized medical departments with full-time physicians were common in larger companies. The railroads were the leading industry to develop extensive employee medical programs. In the early days, railroad lines retained private practitioners along their routes to treat accident cases. They also set up services under full-time chief surgeons. They established claims departments and relief associations to pay for medical expenses and provide minimal support for disabled workers.

For the mining and lumber industries, geographic conditions were the principal reason for extensive company involvement in medical care. Doctors were guaranteed a salary, usually out of

---

[15]Bruce Steinwald and Duncan Neuhauser, "The Role of the Proprietary Hospital," *Law and Contemporary Problems* (Autumn 1970): Table 1, p. 819.

mandatory deductions from workers' wages, as an inducement to move to isolated areas.

Employees' medical programs were also started in some companies as part of a movement known as welfare capitalism. Employers provided a broad range of welfare services, including schools, housing, social and religious programs, and medical care. By 1930 company medical services covered an estimated 540,000 workers in mining and lumbering and approximately 530,000 railway employees and their dependents.[16]

Medical societies, such as the AMA, regarded the corporate doctor as a form of exploitation because the arrangement enabled companies to get doctors to bid against each other and drive down the price of their labor. Consequently, the opposition of the medical profession to the company doctor contributed to the reluctance of employers to expand medical services, and there continued to be tensions between the AMA and company physicians. (In 1908 a physician who had been a company doctor at Sears and Roebuck resigned because the Chicago Medical Society excluded him from membership.)

In the early part of this century prepaid medical insurance developed both in Oregon and in Washington largely as a result of the hazardous working conditions in the lumber, railroad, and mining industries.[17] Typical policies provided for comprehensive medical and hospital care in return for a fixed fee, which was divided between employer and employee. The insurance companies, called hospital associations, were originally begun by physicians but were later managed by nonmedical personnel. Some associations owned their own hospitals, and others used the facilities of community hospitals. Because many of the associations were profit-making institutions, they had excellent incentives to control medical costs.

In the late 19th century fraternal orders and benefits societies became extensively involved in providing life insurance and aiding the sick and disabled. By the early 1900s some 8 million Americans belonged to fraternal orders. Doctors conducted examinations for the life insurance offered by the fraternal orders and began to accept contracts to care for lodge members. So-called lodge practice was

[16]Starr, p. 202.
[17]Ibid., pp. 200–206.

especially common in immigrant communities. A 1917 survey in New York City found thousands of health insurance funds, mostly branches of larger fraternal organizations.[18]

The AMA opposed lodge practice, objecting to the unlimited service for limited pay and the "ruinous competition" it invariably introduced.[19] Many county medical societies refused membership to any doctor who contracted with a lodge.

The evolution in health care in the United States around the turn of the century established the medical profession as we know it by expanding the duties and formal education of physicians and fostering the growth of the hospital system. The first years of the 20th century also witnessed the beginnings of health insurance as a method of prepaying health care costs and the AMA's growing control over the medical marketplace.

The Evolutionary 1930s

A look at the history of health insurance in the United States reveals not the competitive marketplace that most believe exists but an industry filled with the anti-competitive efforts of medical societies and hospitals to suppress alternatives, guarantee their own income, and use government intervention to further their own objectives.

The Great Depression and the Acceptance of Health Insurance

By 1930 the United States had at least as many medical, nursing, and dental schools and hospital beds per unit of population as it has today. The Great Depression, however, slowed the expansion of health care facilities and personnel. Many Americans had severe trouble paying for the medical care they needed. Doctors tried to make allowances for patients in financial straits, but hospitals, with higher fixed costs, had much less flexibility. Between 1929 and 1930 average hospital receipts plummeted from more than $200 per patient to less than $60.[20] Spurred by the ravages of the depression, patients and hospital administrators began to look for some way to

[18]Ibid., pp. 206–9.
[19]"Contract Practice," *Journal of the American Medical Association* 49 (December 14, 1907): 2028–29; and "Contract Practice," *Journal of the American Medical Association* 57 (July 8, 1911): 145–46.
[20]Califano, p. 41.

pay and be paid. Hospitals then began to turn to insurance plans as a way to guarantee a steady cash flow by spreading the financial risk.

The first plan was introduced in 1929 at Baylor University Hospital in Dallas, Texas. A group of 1,500 schoolteachers contracted with the hospital to provide care should they need it in return for a monthly fee paid in advance. The fee was paid whether or not the individual teacher ever used the services. By spreading the risk over a number of teachers, the hospital could afford to provide care if and when it was needed.

The idea caught on, and other hospitals set up similar plans. Soon, groups of nonprofit hospitals in several cities organized multiple-hospital insurance plans. Such plans gave subscribers a choice of medical care providers and thereby attracted more patients and strengthened the income of the participating hospitals. The multiple-hospital plans served as a model for Blue Cross, which was established in 1932 in Sacramento, California.

The multiple-hospital insurance plans changed the concept of insurance and forever changed the American health care system. Unlike other forms of insurance, such as home or automobile, the primary purpose of such plans was not to protect consumers from large, unforeseen expenses but to keep hospitals in business by guaranteeing them a regular income. Although the plans did benefit consumers by giving them a predictable method of paying for their medical care, such plans contained three serious flaws that would become increasingly apparent as the health care system developed.

First, the plans centered on front-end coverage. They would pay for initial hospitalization and then terminate coverage after a specified number of days, thereby exposing patients to high out-of-pocket costs. This feature encouraged hospitalization and contributed to the rise in health care costs.

Second, the plans reinforced the public notion of hospitals as the primary providers of medical care. To take advantage of their hospital plan, patients had to be treated in the hospital. This requirement was a first step toward a medical care system biased in favor of specific providers or services.

Third, the plans established a method for paying health insurance benefits that was different from the way benefits were paid under other forms of insurance. Instead of providing indemnity coverage, hospital plans paid service benefits. Under indemnity plans, such as automobile insurance, policyholders are directly reimbursed a specified amount to compensate for their losses. Under service-benefits policies, the insurance covers certain specified services, whatever their cost may be. Holders of such policies have little incentive to get the best value for their money, and the service providers have every incentive to increase the cost of services or continue recommending additional services of marginal benefit.

The Rise of Blue Cross and Commercial Insurance

In 1932 a community-wide health plan was developed in California. Under it, participating hospitals in a given area agreed to provide services for subscribers, who paid their premiums to the plan rather than to individual hospitals. This concept eliminated any competition among participating hospitals. Hospitals in other areas embraced such plans and marketed them on a not-for-profit basis. They became known as Blue Cross plans. By 1937 these plans had 800,000 subscribers, whereas competing plans set up by individual hospitals had only 125,000.[21] By 1940 membership in Blue Cross plans had ballooned to 6 million.[22]

In response to Blue Cross, commercial insurers began to offer health plans. They calculated rates based on their experience related to differences in age and health. Commercial policies offered cash payments to individuals instead of paying hospitals directly, and coverage was provided for physician services. By 1940 commercial insurers covered 3.7 million people.[23] In response to the expansion of commercial health insurance, doctors established Blue Shield plans to cover physician services.

In the mid-1930s some state insurance commissions tried to subject multiple-hospital plans to the same government regulations as other types of insurance. They wanted to require these new plans to maintain reserve funds—that is, to set aside a portion of their premium revenues to cover unexpectedly large claims. In response, hospitals and doctors, working with the American Hospital Association and the AMA, promoted state legislation to exempt Blue Cross plans from normal insurance regulations. In exchange, Blue Cross

[21]Ibid., pp. 41–42.
[22]Ibid., p. 42.
[23]Ibid.

plans were required to serve the entire community by providing insurance to anyone who wanted it and charging rates that were affordable to low-income people. Blue Cross plans received federal tax exemption as nonprofit organizations and were also often exempted from other taxes, such as real estate taxes. In some states, commercial insurance policies sold to individuals were required to meet minimum benefit/premium rates, whereas Blue Cross policies were not.

The combination of rates negotiated with providers and regulatory exemptions gave Blue Cross enormous financial advantages over other insurers. Of the total population with hospital insurance in 1940, half were covered by Blue Cross, and until the 1980s, Blue Cross and Blue Shield never held less than 40 percent of the entire health insurance market.[24] Unlike other health insurance companies, Blue Cross and Blue Shield were never enemies of the medical community. In fact, many believed that they were created to represent and protect the hospitals and physicians. A majority of the governing boards of both Blue Cross and Blue Shield in 1959 were either hospital trustees or administrators and physicians. Hospital finance experts Howard J. Berman and Lewis B. Weeks concluded, "Blue Cross was founded to save hospitals from financial ruin."[25]

Probably the most interesting and devastating contribution made by the Blues to the health care system consisted of the reimbursement procedures they adopted. Hospitals approved of those procedures, and because of the domination of the market by the Blues, other commercial insurers were forced to adopt the same policies to remain competitive. This reimbursement procedure, known as cost-plus, has contributed significantly to the continued rise in health care costs.

The Problem of Cost-Plus Reimbursement

Under the Blues during the 1930s, physicians were reimbursed either according to a negotiated schedule of fees or on the basis of what insurers considered to be reasonable and customary charges. Hospitals were reimbursed based on the cost-plus method. For

[24]Health Insurance Association of America, *Sourcebook of Health Insurance Data, 1984–1985* (Washington, 1986), Tables 1.2, 1.3, 1.4, and 1.5.

[25]Howard J. Berman and Lewis B. Weeks, *The Financial Management of Hospitals*, 5th ed. (Washington: Health Administration Press, 1982), p. 147.

doctors, that reimbursement scheme meant they would be paid whatever they charged, provided it was generally comparable to the fees charged by other doctors in their locality. For hospitals, cost-plus reimbursement meant that the insurer paid the hospital a percentage of its costs, based on the percentage of policyholders using the hospital's services, plus an additional sum equal to a percentage of the hospital's working and equity capital.

A consequence of this arrangement was the creation of a tremendous incentive for hospitals to increase costs. Under a cost-plus system, increased costs meant additional income for a hospital, whereas reduced costs meant diminished income. The more a hospital improved its facilities, equipment, or services, the more revenue it received. In essence, under the cost-plus system, health insurance companies insured that hospitals had enough income to cover their costs. Insurers came to represent the interests of the hospitals, not those of the purchasers of medical services. Because hospitals and physicians could increase their incomes by increasing their costs, the cost-plus system inevitably led to higher health care costs.

Under the cost-plus system, pressures to increase spending on health care were relentless. Patients had no reason to show restraint in that the money they spent belonged not to them but to a third party. The role of the insurance company in the system was to pay whatever bills were submitted, with few questions asked. Cost increases were then passed along to policyholders in the form of higher health insurance premiums.

Cost-plus reimbursement, now entrenched in the health care system, is contradictory to the operation of a free market, in which prices and competition allocate resources. It frequently creates incentives that are the opposite of those created by the free market. For example, under the free-market system, a surplus of hospital beds would translate into falling prices and a boon for patients. However, under cost-plus, surplus beds mean nothing—except that health care costs will continue to rise. Any additional capital and equipment expenditures (including those for beds) translate into additional reimbursement. Although it appears that a market is functioning in health care and competition is present, what really drives the system goes undetected—cost-plus.[26]

[26]For a more detailed explanation of cost-plus, see John C. Goodman and Gerald Musgrave, *The Changing Market for Health Insurance: Opting Out of the Cost-Plus System*,

The Creation of Prepaid Health Plans

About the same time the first hospital insurance plan was being instituted at Baylor University Hospital, the idea of a prepaid health plan began to emerge. In 1929 employees of the Los Angeles Department of Water and Power arranged with two physicians to provide comprehensive services for about 2,000 workers and their families.[27] The plan cost each subscriber $2 a month and provided hospital and medical care. Soon, other employee groups joined the program, and by 1935 the Ross-Loos Clinic had enrolled more than 12,000 workers and 25,000 dependents.[28]

Five years later Kaiser Industries asked Dr. Sidney Garfield to form a group practice to provide medical services for workers building the Grand Coulee Dam in the state of Washington. In Dallas a mutual benefit association of about 800 street railway workers contracted with a private clinic for medical services; the workers paid 85 cents a month, while the company contributed $100 monthly.[29]

In rural America, groups of consumers organized plans that hired physicians to provide medical care services in return for a fixed salary. Such cooperatives charged their members a predetermined fixed fee. The first so-called medical cooperative, the Farmers Union Hospital Association, was formed in 1929 in Elk City, Oklahoma, by Dr. Michael Shadid. The members owned the hospital, paid staff doctors a fixed salary, and received prepaid medical care.

The AMA was hostile to both prepaid plans and consumer cooperatives, and it launched a campaign to enact legislation that would regulate and even outlaw the plans. Even when prepaid plans were controlled by physicians, the AMA disapproved of them as a form of unethical contract practice. In Los Angeles, for example, the founders of the Ross-Loos Clinic were expelled from their local medical societies. In Oklahoma the local medical profession repeatedly tried to deprive Dr. Shadid of his medical license, frightening away physicians who wanted to join the cooperative and keeping out of the local medical association those physicians who did join.

NCPA Policy Report no. 118 (Dallas: National Center for Policy Analysis, September 1985).

[27]Starr, p. 301.

[28]Ibid.

[29]Ibid., pp. 301–2.

Shadid eventually triumphed in a lawsuit that charged the local medical association with restraint of trade, and physicians in the cooperative were then admitted to membership in the association.

The question of cooperative medicine finally came to a head when the AMA was indicted on charges of violating the Sherman Antitrust Act in its efforts to suppress the Group Health Association of Washington, D.C. GHA was organized in 1937, by employees of the Federal Home Loan Bank, as a nonprofit cooperative to provide medical and hospital care through salaried physicians. Immediately, the AMA called on government authorities to take legal action against what it regarded as unregulated health insurance and the corporate practice of medicine. Unsuccessful in enlisting the government's help, the AMA threatened retaliation against the plan's doctors and persuaded Washington hospitals not to accept the plan. The U.S. Supreme Court upheld a conviction of the AMA on antitrust violations in 1943.

Beginning in 1939 medical associations successfully lobbied for state intervention to ensure professional control of prepayment insurance plans. Within the next decade 26 states passed laws effectively barring consumer-run medical service plans. In those states the incorporators of a medical service plan had to be doctors, or a majority of directors had to be doctors, or the plan had to be approved by the state medical society.

Seventeen states required all plans to allow free choice of physician. Free choice of physician effectively ruled out the prepaid group practice plans. It also prevented plans from including only those doctors and hospitals that might agree to charge a lower price or give better service. And because free choice was feasible in a plan only if the doctors accepted a definite fee schedule, and because only the medical society could provide such a fee schedule (in that plans had to be approved by the state medical society), the requirement for free choice conferred on the medical profession a monopoly in medical service plans. All of the various state restrictions on prepaid medical plans were significant in retarding the growth of such plans and skewing the market toward fee-for-service medical care and indemnity insurance such as that offered by Blue Cross and Blue Shield.

The Growth of Government Health Care Programs

The government's role in providing the public with health care continued to expand during the 1930s. The Ransdell Act, signed in

May 1930, conferred on the National Institutes of Health (NIH) the mandate of ascertaining the cause, prevention, and cure of disease. The following month the NIH Division of Mental Hygiene expanded its mandate to include causes, prevention, and treatment of mental and nervous diseases.

In 1936 Mr. and Mrs. Luke Wilson donated their home and 45 acres in suburban Maryland to the Public Health Service. This property would become the campus of the NIH. Dr. Thomas Parran, selected by President Franklin D. Roosevelt to become surgeon general in 1936, immediately began expansion and modernization of the public health system, and he began grants-in-aid to the states in 1937. Parran expressed the view that "citizens should have an equal opportunity for health as an inherent right with the right of liberty and the pursuit of happiness."[30] He was an advocate of continued expansion of the NIH and also was a founder of the World Health Organization.

In 1938 the Interdepartmental Technical Committee on Medical Care, whose members were from the Public Health Service, the Children's Bureau, and the Social Security Board, proposed a national health program that would include expanded public medical care for all the medically needy and a comprehensive program designed to increase and improve medical service for the entire population, financed by general taxation or by specific insurance contributions from the beneficiaries. In February 1939 Sen. Robert Wagner of New York introduced a national health bill, which incorporated these provisions. But President Roosevelt never pushed for passage of a national health plan, stating that it was "impossible to go up against the medical societies."[31] He was also aware of public opinion polls that showed that Americans still favored a private system of health care.

So, the decade of the 1930s was one of collusion. Physicians and hospitals supported the types of insurance and health care plans that secured their income and worked against the types that didn't,

---

[30]Jesse L. Steinfeld, "The United States Public Health Service," in Department of Health, Education, and Welfare, chap. 5, p. 74.

[31]Starr, p. 279.

oftentimes enlisting the help of government in doing so. The establishment of cost-plus reimbursement, favored by the medical community, was to have far-reaching consequences for the health of the U.S. system of medical care.

The War and Postwar Period (1940–60)

The Growth of Employer-Provided Health Insurance

The major development in health care during the 1940s was the growth of employer-provided health insurance. World War II brought about a shortage of labor, and wartime wage and price controls prohibited employers from increasing salaries to attract workers. However, in 1942 the War Labor Board decided that fringe benefits up to 5 percent of wages would not be considered inflationary. Employers began to offer health benefits as a way of providing additional compensation. Total enrollment in group hospital plans grew from less than 7 million to about 26 million subscribers from 1942 to 1945.[32]

World War II also brought about a major change in taxation. Previously, much of the revenue gathered by the federal government had come from excises and tariffs, with smaller amounts coming from the income tax. However, by the end of the war in 1945, the income tax had surpassed all other sources of revenue for the federal government. The number of Americans filing tax returns in 1940 was 14.6 million; by 1945 that number had risen to 49.8 million—an increase of 350 percent, although the population had increased by only 6 percent.[33] Tax rates rose from 4 percent in 1939 to 23 percent by 1944.[34] The year 1943 saw the permanent institution of the withholding system, under which the government receives tax payments at the front end. Taxes are taken out of a worker's paycheck before it is seen, making them less painful and easier for the government to collect.[35]

---

[32]Starr, p. 311.

[33]Gerald Carson, *"The Golden Egg" The Personal Income Tax: Where It Came from, How It Grew* (Boston: Houghton Mifflin, 1977), pp. 124–29.

[34]Ibid.

[35]There are many who contend that this "out-of-sight, out-of-mind" type of taxation also makes it easier for the government to continually raise taxes, all the time collecting interest on the withheld tax payments.

Concurrently, the Internal Revenue Service (IRS) ruled that the purchase of health insurance for workers was a legitimate cost of doing business and could be deducted from taxable business income. The IRS also ruled that workers did not have to include the value of health insurance benefits in calculating their taxable income. These IRS rulings were a giant tax incentive for both employers and taxpayers, and they did much to institutionalize employer-provided health care as part of the system.

The unions soon recognized that employer-provided health care was a desirable benefit and began to negotiate for it in their contracts. In 1941 Chrysler agreed to set up a group health plan with its recently recognized union. The initial plan covered only hospitalization, and employees paid the entire cost through payroll deductions. The Congress of Industrial Organization declared in 1946 that health insurance was a high priority, and by 1948, 10 unions had negotiated health and welfare plans. That same year the National Labor Relations Board ruled that health benefits were a legitimate subject of collective bargaining, and that finding encouraged the spread of plans even after the end of the war.

In the *Inland Steel* case of 1949, the U.S. Supreme Court ruled that certain fringe benefits, including health care plans, were among the collective bargaining issues that the Taft-Hartley Labor Relations Act gave unions the right to negotiate. The number of union workers covered by health plans rose from 2.7 million in 1949 to 12 million by 1955.[36] Unions, through collective bargaining, became a significant influence on the medical care system.

Collective bargaining agreements expanded the scope of coverage as well as employers' contributions. Coverage of non-hospital medical expenses caught up with insurance against hospital bills. By the end of 1954 over 60 percent of the population had some type of hospital insurance, 50 percent had some type of surgical insurance, and 25 percent had medical insurance.[37] In 1945 employers paid only 10 percent of health care expenses; by 1950, however, collective bargaining agreements were typically requiring them to pay an average of 37 percent. And in 1959 the United Steelworkers

[36]Joseph W. Garbarino, *Health Plans and Collective Bargaining* (Berkeley: University of California Press, 1960), pp. 19–20.

[37]Odin W. Anderson and Jacob J. Feldman, *Family Medical Costs and Voluntary Health Insurance: A Nationwide Survey* (New York: McGraw-Hill, 1956), p. 11.

ended a 116-day strike when a settlement was reached that required the steel companies to pay the entire premium for health insurance. General Motors, the Ford Motor Company, and the Chrysler Corporation followed with similar agreements with the United Automobile Workers in 1961.

An entirely new system of health care financing was created during the 1940s and 1950s. Government encouraged the development and expansion of provider-oriented insurance plans that ultimately distorted the health care delivery system. Employer-provided plans offering first-dollar, routine-care coverage contributed significantly to the rise in health care costs. The inflationary effect of third-party payment, attributable to the preponderance of employer-provided insurance, worsened the position of those without health plans. Pressure from those left out of the system resulted in government's intervening with its own health programs.

The Flaws of First-Dollar Coverage

Health insurance policies that cover first-dollar expenses (front-end coverage) pay for routine care. The defect in most of these policies is that there is no coverage for the medical calamities that will economically wipe out patients and their families. Interestingly, front-end health insurance operates contrary to all other forms of insurance. The most obvious example is automobile insurance; drivers insure themselves against catastrophic damage and loss but pay out-of-pocket for routine repairs and maintenance.

Policies that pay for routine care actually favor the interests of physicians and hospitals more than those of patients. Under routine (acute-care) plans, the more treatment doctors or hospitals provide, the more money they receive. Under such plans, doctors are encouraged to prescribe additional treatments up to the limit of the patient's insurance coverage, even though the treatments may improve the patient's health or well-being only slightly.

Why do people purchase first-dollar, routine-care coverage for their health care when they wouldn't think of purchasing such coverage for their automobile? Simply stated, they do so because the tax code encourages them to do so. Health insurance plans are viewed as tax-free compensation, not as real insurance. Workers favor coverage that pays for routine care, freeing their discretionary income for other uses. Insurance is no longer used for its normal purpose of spreading risk but for tax avoidance.

This form of coverage influences patients to demand additional and possibly unnecessary medical services because they have no reason to question the costs. Doctors and hospitals do not have any financial incentives to control costs either, and therefore they increase the prices and quantity of their services. Insurance companies, which normally keep a percentage of claims costs, also have little incentive to control services.

Besides enacting tax incentives that skewed the insurance market, government intervention generated another problem in the industry in the 1940s: experience rating. Because the government protected the Blues by exempting them from taxes and reserve requirements, those companies had a competitive advantage over commercial insurers. Consequently, commercial insurers turned to experience rating their insurance plans as a way of competing against the Blues.

Usually, insurance companies use some form of community rating to calculate a basic premium. The premium reflects the average frequency and cost of claims among all the policyholders in a given area. Under an experience-rating system, though, the cost of the premium depends on the actual experience of individual policyholders and is based on the frequency and size of the claims they file. Commercial insurers began to sell insurance to employers with relatively healthy, low-risk employees at cheaper rates than the Blues. Because the Blues often were required by law to use a community-rating system, they responded to this competition by requesting, and receiving, permission to use a modified community rating to reflect experience.

The problem evolved that companies calculated premiums for group plans on the basis of people who worked for a single employer. As a result, smaller companies that had fewer employees over whom to spread costs generally paid more for insurance. In addition, they faced the risk of large premium increases or even cancellation if even one employee became ill. Had the government not intervened on behalf of the Blues and provided them with legislative protection, commercial insurers may not have developed the experience-rating system in order to compete. That system, still in operation, has resulted in a significant portion of small businesses being unable to afford health insurance coverage for their employees.

The Surge in Government Health Programs

World War II sparked a great expansion of the federal government's role in health care. There were four major postwar health programs: medical research, mental health, the Veterans' Administration, and hospital construction.

In 1939 the Public Health Service operated a wide array of medical services for merchant seamen, prison inmates, Coast Guardsmen, lepers, and narcotics addicts, and its mandate continued to expand. It administered public health grants to the states and special programs of state grants for the control of venereal disease and tuberculosis. The war gave medical research priority, and in July 1941 President Roosevelt created the Office of Scientific Research and Development, with two committees on national defense and medical research.

The NIH budget was beginning to swell. Between 1945 and 1947 its research budget expanded from $180,000 to $4 million.[38] By 1950 this budget had grown to $46.3 million.[39] Like other health organizations, the NIH discovered that the way to acquire money from Congress was to call attention to one disease at a time. In 1948 Congress created a National Heart Institute, and soon five other institutes followed. In 1950 Congress established the National Science Foundation, and in 1953 it created the Department of Health, Education, and Welfare.

Funds for medical research rose at a dramatic pace starting at the outset of the war. Between 1941 and 1951 the federal budget for medical research rose from $3 million to $76 million.[40] Between 1955 and 1960 the NIH budget exploded from $81 million to $400 million.[41]

The fastest growing of the various divisions of the NIH was the National Institute of Mental Health. Between 1948 and 1962 NIMH research grants rose from $374,000 to $42.6 million.[42] Under its

[38]Starr, p. 342.

[39]Starr, p. 343.

[40]Kenneth M. Endicott and Ernest M. Allen, "The Growth of Medical Research 1941–1953 and the Role of the Public Health Service Research Grants," *Science* 118 (September 25, 1953): 337.

[41]Congressional Quarterly Service, *Congress and the Nation, 1945–1964*, vol. 1, p. 1132.

[42]Starr, p. 346.

broad mandate, the agency's research programs included child development, juvenile delinquency, suicide prevention, alcoholism, and television violence.

By World War II the Veterans' Administration had 91 institutions and ran the largest hospital system in the country. Following the war the VA built new hospitals in urban areas and established close affiliations with medical schools. There were about 71,000 veterans hospitalized in August 1945; and by May 1946 this number had risen to 86,000 and soon increased to 105,000.[43] Nearly 16 million new veterans returned home to the United States after World War II. The VA medical staff increased from 2,300 doctors in June 1945 to 4,000 in June 1946.[44]

During and after the war, the government became more deeply involved in hospital construction. In 1942 the American Hospital Association organized the Commission on Hospital Care to lobby for a national program of hospital construction. Three private foundations (the Kellogg Foundation, the Commonwealth Foundation, and the National Foundation for Infantile Paralysis)—plus the Public Health Service—provided financial and staff support. The commission recommended a huge program of construction: an additional 195,000 beds at an investment of $1.8 billion. In 1946 the Hospital Survey and Construction Act (the Hill-Burton Act) was passed by Congress. By the time the law expired in 1978, the program had used $4.4 billion in federal money as leverage to get state and local governments to contribute $9.1 billion more, building 500,000 beds.

The period 1940–60 saw expansion of the use of first-dollar coverage health insurance. World War II and tax incentives did much to stimulate the growth of employer-provided insurance plans. The flawed insurance plans conceived in the 1930s planted the seeds of the cost increases that took root during this period.

The Expansionary 1960s

In the 1960s prices in general began to soar. There was an explosion in government programs, legislation, and health care costs.

[43]*Health in America 1776–1976* (Washington: Department of Health, Education, and Welfare, 1976), p. 102.
[44]Ibid., p. 103.

The Explosion in Government Health Legislation

The preponderance of employer-provided health care accentuated the medical needs of those without insurance, primarily the unemployed, poor, and elderly. In the early 1960s pressures began to build for some sort of government health program that would provide care for these groups. In 1960 Congress responded by passing the legislation known as Kerr-Mills. It extended federal support for welfare medicine programs to the states, with the federal government providing between 50 and 80 percent of the funds. But by 1963 the five large industrial states with only 32 percent of the population over 65 were receiving 90 percent of the funds. Proponents began to look for a more effective alternative.

Concern about a doctor shortage began to arise. Politicians equated lack of access with lack of supply. When the AMA countered that there was no shortage, Congress accused it of trying to control the supply of physicians for economic reasons. The AMA responded that the government was interfering with the practice of medicine. Eventually, the government proceeded with a series of initiatives intended to increase supply. The Health Professions Education Assistance Act of 1963 provided construction funds and capitation grants to encourage medical schools to increase the size of their classes. Public Law 89–290, enacted in 1964, created medical scholarships and supplied funds to support the operating costs of schools.

The government programs that would soon follow, such as Medicare and Medicaid, compounded the shortage problem by dramatically increasing the demand for services. In 1964 the nonpoor saw physicians about 20 percent more frequently than the poor; by 1975 the poor visited physicians 18 percent more often than the nonpoor.[45] In 1963 those with incomes under $2,000 a year had only half as many surgical procedures per 100 people as those with incomes of $7,500 or more, but by 1970 the rate for the low-income group was 40 percent higher.[46] In *America's Health Care Revolution*, Joseph Califano, a domestic policy adviser in the Johnson administration, commented on mistakes made during the 1960s:

[45]Karen Davis and Cathy Schoen, *Health and the War on Poverty* (Washington: Brookings Institution, 1978), p. 41.

[46]Ibid., Table 2–8, p. 48.

> Anticipating sharply increased demand for health care ser-
> vices, we pushed through Congress laws to train more doc-
> tors and nurses, build more hospitals, and set up commu-
> nity health centers. The assumption was that we were play-
> ing by traditional economic rules: the more doctors and
> hospitals, the more competition, the more efficient and less
> costly the services. By 1967 and 1968 we realized how mis-
> guided this assumption was. The rise of health care costs
> was accelerating dramatically.[47]

Dissatisfied with a piecemeal approach, people who had champi-
oned the New Deal programs of the 1930s began agitating anew for
a national health plan, while groups such as the AMA, which
feared adoption of such a program, advocated decentralized, state-
administered programs that would maintain the autonomy of physicians and hospitals. A compromise was reached in 1965, and the
Medicare program was born.

With this legislation, Congress declared that a minimum level of
health care was the right of every U.S. citizen. Medicare, through
an intermediary (usually Blue Cross), provided direct payment for
the care of the elderly. The largest portion of the program, Medicare
Part A, Hospital Insurance, was a slimmed-down version of the
universal social insurance scheme advocated by proponents of
national health insurance. The other section, Medicare Part B, Supplemental Medical Insurance, was a voluntary program to cover
physician services with a mixture of premiums and general federal
revenues.

Medicaid was based on the alternative originally proposed by the
AMA. Financed by a combination of matching federal and state
funds and administered by the states, it paid for medical care for
the poor, regardless of age. In an instant, with the passage of
Medicare and Medicaid, the government had become the largest
single purchaser of health care.

With the adoption of Medicare and Medicaid, the third-party
payment system dominated the health care industry. Most Americans' hospital and physician costs were covered either by private
health insurance or a government program. But Medicare and Medicaid brought the defects found in the private insurance industry

[47]Califano, p. 53.

to the entire health care landscape, dramatically accelerating the rate of medical price inflation already set in motion by cost-plus reimbursement, lack of patient incentive to control costs, and first-dollar coverage.

The cost-plus reimbursement policies of private insurance were replicated in Medicare and also by many states in their Medicaid programs. Hospitals charged Medicare for the "reasonable cost" of treating patients, and doctors were reimbursed for their "reasonable and customary" fees. According to Califano, federal adoption of the cost-based, fee-for-service reimbursement system became a blank check for American hospitals and doctors. The volume of hospital services reimbursed on a cost-plus basis rose 75 percent as a result of Medicare and Medicaid. The rate of increase in hospital spending, which had averaged 8.8 percent between 1960 and 1965, almost doubled, approaching an average annual increase of 15 percent from 1965 to 1970. Sharp rises occurred in hospital staffing, wages, and the purchase of new equipment and supplies.[48] These cost increases were driven by increased utilization and by demands for pay increases by hospital staff who appreciated that the government, rather than the patient, was now paying.

Medicare's benefit structure favored the same kind of first-dollar, routine coverage as private insurance. Under Medicare Part A, patients were charged a small deductible but paid nothing else for a 60-day hospital stay. After 60 days, Medicare paid a decreasing amount, saddling seriously ill patients with catastrophic costs.

The medical care provided for beneficiaries under Medicare and Medicaid was either free or greatly subsidized, and premiums were nonexistent or unrelated to individual or group usage. Consequently, beneficiaries had no incentive to question costs and every motivation to demand more services.

Problems with Physicians and Hospitals

Besides endowing the Medicare program with the same defects and flaws found in the private insurance industry, the federal government added insult to injury when it came to writing the regulations involving physician and hospital reimbursement for Medicare patients.

[48]Ibid., pp. 54–55.

WHAT HAS GOVERNMENT DONE TO OUR HEALTH CARE?

Following the passage of Medicare, the Johnson administration was faced with threats from physicians and hospitals that they would not participate in the program. In response to White House pressure to get the plan off to a running start, the Department of Health, Education, and Welfare wrote regulations regarding reimbursement that were extremely beneficial to the medical industry. Not only did doctors get the power to charge so-called reasonable and customary fees, they also were given significant control over how Medicare would set such fees.

Hospitals were successful in getting the interest on current and capital debt included in reimbursement costs and pressured HEW to pay for depreciation on buildings and equipment that had been purchased with federal funds under the Hill-Burton Act. In addition, government officials agreed to give hospitals a 2 percent add-on to their actual costs for treating Medicare patients. According to Joseph Califano, "The 2 percent was a bribe to get the hospital industry to cooperate with Medicare."[49] The decision to provide capital reimbursement under Medicare involved millions of dollars annually in federal expenditures over and above the monies spent through the Hill-Burton program.

Additional Government Health Care Programs

Other government programs providing health care services, usually to specific populations within the country, witnessed a significant increase in services and costs starting in the 1960s. The programs included those of the Public Health Service, the Indian Health Service, the armed services, and the former Veterans' Administration.

The arm of the Public Health Service (PHS) reached into new health concerns during this period. It established a program for the detection and treatment of hypertension. The surgeon general completed a report associating television watching with anti-social behavior. Surgeon general reports detailing the ills of smoking began to appear. The PHS established a National Institute on Alcoholism and a family planning and population growth program. In 1955 it took over responsibility for the Indian Health Service from

[49]Ibid., p. 144.

the Department of the Interior. By 1989 the annual outlays for the PHS totaled approximately $85 billion.[50]

The Indian Health Service provides health care and public health services to approximately 1 million Native Americans through a network of hospitals and clinics. By 1989 the service's annual outlays were approximately $1.9 billion.[51]

The Department of Defense (DoD) runs its own health care system for members and retirees of the armed forces and their dependents, approximately 10 million people, at an annual cost of around $9 billion.[52] DoD operates 165 hospitals as well as hundreds of clinics.

The number of veterans aged 65 and over being treated by the Department of Veterans' Affairs will grow from approximately 7.2 million in 1990 to 10 million in 2000. The health care bill, which totaled $10 billion in 1989 and $30 billion in 1990, could rise to $50 billion by the year 2000.[53] The VA operates 172 medical centers and hospitals with 80,000 beds, 233 outpatient clinics, 122 nursing homes with 9,000 beds, and 16 veterans' homes, plus a variety of programs for home care and geriatric day and resident care.[54] It employs about 240,000 medical workers. Unlike Medicare, the VA charges no premiums, copayments, or deductibles. There have been some attempts in the past to modify the VA health care system for cost-containment reasons, but because care of the veteran is such a political issue, those attempts have as yet been unsuccessful.

Block grant programs used by the federal government to provide health care services to various populations include the Maternal and Child Health Block Grant program (the 1992 estimated budget is $554 million, up from $373 million in 1982); the Preventive Health and Health Services Block Grant program (the 1992 estimated budget is $150 million, up from $92.5 million in 1981); and the Alcohol,

---

[50]The Budget for Fiscal Year 1991, Department of Health and Human Services, Public Health Service Management, p. A–715.

[51]Ibid., p. A–696.

[52]Califano, p. 158.

[53]Ibid., p. 156.

[54]Ibid.

Drug Abuse, and Mental Health Block Grant program (the 1992 estimated budget is $1.3 billion, up from $543 million in 1981).[55]

The 1960s were a decade of vast expansion by the government into the area of health care. The rise in health care prices during this period was really a prelude to what was to come—the cost explosions and regulatory mood of the 1970s and 1980s.

The Regulatory 1970s and 1980s

The eruption in health care costs over the past few decades has been staggering. Personal health care expenditures increased from $82 per capita in 1950 to $1,837 per capita in 1986.[56] By the year 2000 the health care bill is expected to top $5,510 for each man, woman, and child in the United States.[57]

The Cost Explosion in Health Care

Spiraling medical costs have strained government programs. Between 1978 and 1988, Medicare spending jumped from $25.2 billion to $87.6 billion, a growth in constant dollars of 99 percent.[58] At the same time, total Medicaid program expenses rose from $18.9 billion in 1978 to $54.7 billion in 1988, a 65 percent increase in constant dollars.[59]

The higher inflation rates of the 1970s exacerbated the weaknesses in the health care financing system. As prices increased, workers demanded higher wages, which often pushed those workers into higher tax brackets. Rising tax liability made employer-provided nontaxable benefits, such as health care plans, increasingly more attractive. More companies began to offer health insurance plans to workers, and unions demanded additional benefit coverage to make up for a loss in disposable income. For example, between 1970 and

---

[55]From Cindi Berry, legislative assistant for health care issues for Rep. Jon Kyl (R-Ariz.). She received the information from personal correspondence with other government officials.

[56]David Holzman, "Medicine Minus a Cost Tourniquet," *Insight*, August 8, 1988.

[57]Jack Meyer, Sean Sullivan, and Sharon Silow-Carroll, *Critical Choices: Confronting the Cost of American Health Care*, report by New Direction for Policy for the Naional Committee for Quality Health Care (Washington, 1990), p. 32.

[58]Committee on Ways and Means, U.S. House of Representatives, *Background Material and Data on Programs within the Jurisdiction of the Committee on Ways and Means*, 1989 ed., March 15, 1989, pp. 1140–41.

[59]Ibid., pp. 152, 1139–40.

1980 the number of Americans with dental insurance plans rose from 12 million to 80 million.[60]

The ability to exclude health insurance from taxable income encourages employees to purchase too much insurance for their needs. John Goodman has made the argument that for a highly paid employee (facing a 6 percent state and local income tax rate), $1.97 in wages is equivalent to $1 in health insurance.[61] This fact encourages employees to prefer overly generous (and wasteful) health insurance coverage— coverage they would not buy out of pocket without tax incentives. For a highly paid employee, $1.97 spent on health insurance need only be worth $1.01 to be preferable to $1.97 in wages. If that money is paid in wages, the employee will be left with just $1 of take-home pay. Moreover, since highly paid workers tend to dictate the contents of employee benefits plans, their choices are extended to all other workers.[62]

The tax law also encourages overinsurance by allowing doctors' fees to be paid by an employer with pretax dollars, whereas fees paid by employees must come from after-tax dollars. This arrangement encourages first-dollar, low-deductible health coverage. Insurance that covers small medical bills has proven to be the most wasteful, as it usually costs an insurance company more than $50 to administer and monitor a claim for a $50 fee, thereby effectively doubling the cost of health care.[63]

During the 1970s and 1980s corporations and small businesses alike began to see their health costs shoot through the roof. A survey of *Fortune* 500 companies and the nation's 250 largest nonindustrial firms found that "from 1981 to 1983, the average rate of increase of health insurance premiums was a staggering 20 percent."[64] Total health care costs for those firms, on average, amounted to 24 percent of after-tax profits.[65] Between 1983 and 1984 medical costs for many corporations

[60]Health Insurance Association of America, *Sourcebook of Health Insurance Data, 1984–1985* (Washington, 1986), Table 1.8.

[61]National Center for Policy Analysis, *An Agenda for Solving America's Health Care Crisis: A Task Force Report* (Dallas, 1990), p. 15.

[62]Ibid.

[63]Ibid.

[64]Regina E. Herzlinger and Jeffrey Schwartz, "How Companies Tackle Health Care Costs: Part I," *Harvard Business Review*, July/August 1985, p. 69.

[65]Ibid.

jumped 20 to 25 percent.[66] American businesses spent $110.5 billion on health insurance premiums in 1988, 40 percent of their pretax profits.[67] That rise meant that large corporations needed to find ways to cut expenses and tighten controls. The increase in health costs usually meant that small businesses had to cut back coverage or cancel policies for their employees.

The experience of the Chrysler Corporation is similar to that of much of corporate America. Despite efforts at cost control, the company's bill for health care in 1984 was $400 million.[68] Adding in Chrysler's share of the Medicare payroll tax and other health insurance premiums brought the total cost by 1989 to more than $700 for each car sold.[69] That was almost 10 times the $75 a car that health care had cost Chrysler in 1970.[70]

Spiraling Malpractice and the Contribution to Rising Costs

Another consequence of the third-party payment system (besides increased demand for services and lack of concern for the cost of procedures) is patients' high expectations for quality care. The results are reflected in the explosion in malpractice lawsuits and the spiraling cost of malpractice insurance.

In the late 19th century several court decisions held that physicians needed only to meet the standard of care of the local communities in which they practiced to avoid liability for malpractice. Early in the 20th century physicians organized malpractice funds for legal defense, and most doctors won their lawsuits.

As the standards for medical care were nationalized, lawsuits became a method of ensuring that every conceivable test or procedure had been done. The plethora of diagnostic tests that accompanied the increased quality of care and cost insulation of the patient by the third-party payment system not only increased health care costs but also gave rise to a standard by which to measure all physicians. Once a physician was found to be negligent in performing a test, the jury was ready to award a sizable judgment.

[66]Califano, p. 164.

[67]Hilary Stout, "Health Costs," *Wall Street Journal*, April 12, 1991.

[68]Califano, p. 30.

[69]Kenneth H. Bacon, "Business and Labor Reach a Consensus on Need to Reduce Health-Care Costs," *Wall Street Journal*, November 1, 1989.

[70]Based on Califano, p. 30.

These events set up a merry-go-round in rising health care costs. The rise in malpractice suits caused doctors and hospitals to order every test that might be significant. Such testing wasn't that onerous in that patients weren't paying for it, but the result was increasing costs. And malpractice insurance premiums began to skyrocket, costing doctors $3.7 billion and hospitals $2 billion by 1985.[71]

An old country saying reflects the state in which Americans were finding the health care system they had created over this century: "The chickens have come home to roost." In the course of the 20th century the health care system had become a morass of government programs and private health insurance riddled with built-in inflationary features. Adding to the problem were the increasing numbers of workers, poor, and elderly priced out of the health care market by these built-in cost increases. Out of frustration, rumbles of support for some kind of national health insurance started to resurface as people searched for a solution.

What Did the Federal Government Do?

As costs continued to escalate through the 1970s and 1980s, what did the federal government do to rectify the situation? Did it rescind its protection of the third-party payment system? Did it remove the tax incentives that encouraged employer-provided insurance? Did it eliminate inflationary policies from the Medicare program? Did it pass legislation nullifying the many laws and restrictions imposed on the health care market? Did it attempt to remove the incentives that result in increased demand for medical care with little concern for the cost?

The answer to all those questions is no. Instead of removing the controls and restrictions that were hampering the market, the federal government attempted to stifle the outcome of bad policies with a whole host of new controls and regulations, like putting so many Band-Aids on a mortal wound. The focus of all the legislation in recent years has been on controlling medical prices and holding down costs, specifically by applying restrictions to physicians, hospitals, and even patients.

Health Maintenance Organizations

Health maintenance organizations (HMOs) were given their official name on February 5, 1970, by Dr. Paul Ellwood in his suite at

[71]Meyer, Sullivan, and Silow-Carroll, p. 59.

the Dupont Plaza in Washington, D.C. Ellwood, a consultant for the Nixon administration, formulated the idea of the HMO as an answer to rising health care costs. His work culminated in the Health Maintenance Organization Act of 1973, which encouraged the development of HMOs as an alternative to traditional insurance plans. HMO physicians are usually salaried employees of an organization that provides its subscribers with medical care for a prepaid fixed fee. HMO managers have an incentive to keep the organization profitable by requiring doctors to be careful about costs and by limiting the freedom of patients to demand services or choose a particular doctor. They also attempt to keep costs down by focusing on preventive medicine.

There were several obstacles to the creation of HMOs, including patient and physician dislike of the lack of choice in care, difficulty in obtaining the necessary start-up capital to establish an HMO, and many state laws supported by medical societies that prohibited the "corporate practice of medicine."

The 1973 act changed this situation by preempting state laws restricting the development of HMOs and by providing HMOs with federal grants and loans as capital. The act also included a significant amount of regulation, including requiring all companies with 25 or more employees to offer an HMO plan to their workers. As a result of the new legislation, the grants and loans, and employers' interest in controlling health care costs, HMOs grew from 26 plans with about 3 million subscribers nationwide in the early 1970s to nearly 700 plans with 28 million enrollees in 1987.[72]

Although the growth of HMOs has been astronomical and some cost containment has been achieved, some physicians are expressing dissatisfaction with HMOs and other managed-care plans (see Chapter 2), and they are questioning the solvency of some of the plans. It must be remembered, too, that although the HMO has been touted as a market-type solution, it was created and financially encouraged by the government, and it continues to be heavily regulated. The severe regulatory and possible financial difficulties faced by HMOs make future efforts to find other market alternatives attractive.

[72]Stuart M. Butler and Edmund F. Haislmaier, eds., *Critical Issues: A National Health System for America* (Washington: Heritage Foundation, 1989), p. 21.

Professional Standards Review Organizations

The original Medicare law mandated that the medical staff of a hospital had to have a utilization review program in order for the hospital to be paid for services to patients. The committee of physicians was to review the appropriateness of admission and the length of stay of every patient. This review was often second-guessed by the insurance company or state agency. Payment was frequently denied, and doctors, hospitals, and patients were dissatisfied.

In response to complaints, Congress introduced professional standards review organizations (PSROs) in 1972. Doctors review their peers' work to ensure that the services that Medicare paid for were medically necessary, were provided according to professional standards, and were rendered at the appropriate level and length of hospital stay. Although there are numerous PSROs in effect today, they have done little to check the rise in doctors' fees or to trim the number or length of hospital stays.[73]

National Health Planning and Resources Development Act

The National Health Planning and Resources Development Act, passed in 1974, attempted to prevent the duplication or overexpansion of health care facilities. The idea was to control capital investment in new facilities and technological equipment, in hopes that the limitation of resources would slow utilization and curb the escalation of costs. The law required states to enact certificate-of-need legislation to implement this kind of control. But the huge bureaucracy of health service agencies that resulted from the law created such a monster that the program ended up costing more than it saved. It was eliminated in 1986 by an act of Congress.

Certificate of Need

Before the federal government required the states to enact certificate-of-need legislation in 1974, many states already required medical institutions, usually both hospitals and nursing homes, to get state approval for construction projects and other large capital investments. Although the states vested authority for such projects in state boards and commissions, they often gave local planning councils an advisory role in the review process. The interest of the

[73]Goodman, pp. 124–28.

state governments was cost control; governments believed hospital beds would be used to the extent they were available.

Prospective Payment System and Diagnostic Related Groups of Illnesses

In 1983 a major effort at controlling Medicare costs was a provision within social security legislation that established a prospective payment system (PPS) for hospital reimbursement. Under this system, Medicare establishes a fixed schedule of fees that it pays hospitals for the treatment of each of 475 diagnostic related groups (DRGs) of illnesses. If the actual cost to the hospital is less than the DRG fee, the hospital keeps the difference; if more, it absorbs the loss. The purpose is to encourage price consciousness and competition among hospitals.

What may have looked good on paper, however, was disappointing in reality. The PPS was destined to cause the same shortages and misallocations that any price control system would cause, and it did so by shifting costs to activities not covered by the controls. Limits on reimbursement amounts for medical treatments covered by Medicare forced hospitals that were losing money on those procedures to make up the difference on other items and treatments. Newspaper and other media stories questioned why a hospital would charge a patient $7 for an aspirin. Cost shifting, attributable to the PPS, was partly to blame.

Not surprisingly, costs in the Medicare program continued to rise. In the first five years after the introduction of the PPS, the average annual rates of growth in Medicare spending were 6.5 percent for the Hospital Insurance program and 13.8 percent for the Supplemental Medical Insurance program, much higher than the overall rate of inflation.[74] Medicare, whose annual program costs were initially estimated at around $5 billion in 1965, had 1990 costs of approximately $111.2 billion.[75]

The expense to private payers from this cost shifting is substantial. The Health Insurance Association of America (HIAA) has estimated that shifted costs jumped from $5.8 billion in 1982 to $8.8

[74]Based on data from the Committee on Ways and Means, p. 152.

[75]"Expenditures for Health Services and Supplies under Public Programs, by Type of Expenditure and Program: 1990," *Health Care Financing Review*, Fall 1991, Table 13, p. 53.

billion in 1984. In its testimony before the Joint Economic Commit-tee, the HIAA remarked that "hospitals recoup reductions in Medi-care and Medicaid reimbursement by inflating charges to private patients. Those who are insured face higher premiums. Those who are not are faced with a ruinous hidden tax exacted at a time when they are least able to pay."[76]

Another form of cost shifting occurs within the PPS. When the cost of treating a patient exceeds Medicare's fixed payment, the result is a form of dumping, in which the patient is transferred to another facility or is discharged early. This procedure has created a two-tier health care system in which those on Medicare receive a lower standard of care.

State Mandated-Benefit Laws

Another piece of regulation that drives up the cost of health care and that is found in a number of states consists of mandated-benefit laws. Usually enacted as a result of lobbying by health care providers and advocates seeking coverage for various diseases, mandated-benefit laws require insurance companies to pay for spe-cific medical services. In 1970 there were only 30 state mandated-benefit laws in the entire country; today there are at least 800.[77] These laws provide a secure market for the providers of the man-dated benefits, with the usual result of increasing demand for the service, increasing providers of the service, and increasing prices.

The laws are also a major reason many people lack health insur-ance. State-mandated benefits increase the cost of insurance and price many people out of the insurance market. According to a study by the National Center for Policy Analysis, as many as one of every four uninsured people lack health insurance because state regulations have increased the price.[78] Consequently, as many as 9.3 million people lack health insurance because of current govern-ment policies.[79]

[76]Quoted in Califano, p. 165.

[77]National Center for Policy Analysis, p. 19.

[78]Ibid.

[79]John C. Goodman and Gerald L. Musgrave, *Freedom of Choice in Health Insurance*, NCPA Policy Report no. 134 (Dallas: National Center for Policy Analysis, November 1988), p. 20.

73

Regulations and Health Care Costs

Regulations involving the approval of drugs and medical devices by the Food and Drug Administration (FDA) have contributed to increased health care costs. In 1962 amendments to the Food, Drug, and Cosmetic Act mandated that new drugs had to be tested and shown to be safe and effective before they were allowed on the market. Since then the process by which a new drug receives approval from the FDA has become increasingly complicated, lengthy, and costly. In 1965 it took approximately two years for FDA approval; by 1989 the time had risen to three years and the cost had increased from about $4 million to over $231 million.[80] In July 1980 the Medical Device Amendments applied some of the same standards to medical devices.

In addition to the health care-related regulations mentioned above, there are numerous government requirements that are not directly related to health care but have an impact on the price of medical care. One obvious example is minimum-wage laws that require health care providers to pay employees a certain wage. Such laws contribute to increased costs as well as lower rates of employment. Another consists of the regulations imposed by the Occupational Safety and Health Administration, which requires certain safety standards in the workplace and enforces them with fines and penalties. The cost to health care providers of complying with such regulations results in significant price increases for medical services.[81]

What Has Business Done?

Faced with mounting health care costs, companies have been forced to adopt cost-control measures. Some corporations offer plans that require an increased contribution from the worker in the form of higher deductibles and coinsurance. Many companies have adopted HMO or other managed-care plans or have taken direct control of their existing plans.

---

[80]Data from correspondence with the Pharmaceutical Manufacturers Association.

[81]Comments on the effects of the regulators of specific government agencies on the cost of health care are summarized from a conversation with Dr. Phillips Gausewitz, president of Pathology Medical Laboratories in San Diego, California.

Self-insurance has been another way some corporations have increased their control over employee health care costs while avoiding state-mandated benefit laws. Some companies offer cafeteria or flexible-benefit plans, under which workers can choose from among a set of company-approved insurance plans and HMOs. Employees who choose less-expensive plans are permitted to select additional nonhealth benefits or are paid increased cash wages.

A few corporations offer year-end cash bonuses to employees who remain healthy and do not use their health insurance. Some workers are offered bonuses for successfully monitoring their medical bills for overcharges. And many corporations, attempting to reduce use of medical care, have instituted wellness programs that educate employees on staying healthy.

Conclusion

Despite the best efforts of business and the best intentions of government, health care costs are still rising and are out of control. The problem remains: until we change the fundamental defects in the system, no amount of tinkering will result in a significant slowing or reversal of increasing costs.

The government's hodgepodge of health care programs, its continual interference in the market, and the protection of its (and the medical community's) preferred methods of care have distorted the market and created a built-in structure of cost escalation. Government is swiftly bringing this country's health care system to the brink of disaster.

4. The Drift toward Nationalized Health Care

The United States is often criticized for being the only industrialized country other than South Africa that lacks a national system of health care. Protection against the costs of sickness became the responsibility of most European governments as long ago as the late 19th century. In 1883 Germany established the first national system of compulsory sickness insurance. Similar systems were adopted in Austria in 1888 and in Hungary in 1891. Compulsory sickness insurance plans were set up in Norway in 1909, in Serbia in 1910, in Britain in 1911, in Russia in 1912, and in the Netherlands in 1913. Other countries, including France, Italy, Sweden, Denmark, and Switzerland, gave state aid to voluntary funds and provided incentives for membership. Political instability and labor unrest during this time period are normally cited as reasons for the passage of national health care programs in several of these countries.

In the United States, however, the political climate for a system of nationalized health care or mandatory insurance has been different from that experienced in Europe. Unlike European countries, which operated under monarchies of one sort or another that applied a paternalistic hand to governing, the United States was formed as a limited-government democracy, in which individual responsibility for almost every area of life was paramount. The idea that government should be responsible for the health of its citizens was foreign and suspect to most Americans.

Recently, a seemingly unusual coalition of interest groups has formed to lobby for a nationalized health care system for the United States. The coalition seems unusual because some members, most notably business and physicians' organizations, are perceived as being historically opposed to any kind of national system. But a quick look at the history of the national health care movement in

America shows that this contemporary coalition is really not that unusual.

The National Health Care Movement in America

In the early part of the 20th century, advocates of nationalized health care in the United States came from both inside and outside the government. In 1904 the Socialist party became the first American political party to endorse national health insurance. The American Association of Labor Legislation (AALL) took up the banner for national health insurance in 1906. In the years preceding World War I, the AALL was successful in encouraging the American Medical Association (AMA) to help formulate a model health insurance bill. President Woodrow Wilson's Commission on Industrial Relations recommended national health insurance in its final report in 1916. Around the same time, the labor committee of the U.S. House of Representatives held hearings on a resolution, introduced by its sole Socialist party member, to create a national social insurance commission.

Support for and opposition to national health insurance came from some unusual places. In 1916 a committee of the National Association of Manufacturers (NAM), a business association, reported that voluntary insurance would be the "higher and better method," but it recognized that compulsory insurance might be necessary and, if so, all occupations ought to be included.[1] Later, however, the NAM came to oppose compulsory health insurance. At the same time, Samuel Gompers and his American Federation of Labor stridently opposed national health insurance, stating that it would create a system of state supervision of the people's health.[2]

The entrance of America into World War I in 1917 turned attention elsewhere, and the movement for national health care waned. One referendum on health insurance took place in California in 1918, with the Social Insurance Commission proposing an amendment to the state constitution. However, a coalition of doctors and religious groups mounted a campaign against the measure, equating it with Germany's social insurance system and arousing wartime anti-German sentiment. The referendum went down in a landslide defeat.

[1] Paul Starr, *The Social Transformation of American Medicine* (New York: Basic Books, 1982), p. 250.
[2] Ibid., p. 249.

Other efforts were made in New York, Ohio, and Pennsylvania, but all were defeated. The end of World War I and the boom of the 1920s sent thoughts of national health insurance to the back of everyone's mind.

During the late 1920s a rise in the costs of medical care prompted the formation of a privately funded commission, the Committee on the Costs of Medical Care. The committee included economists, physicians, and public health specialists. The final report of the committee called for the promotion of group practice and group payment for medical care but opposed compulsory health insurance. The AMA violently opposed the report's recommendations on group practice and payment. So strong was the controversy that when President Franklin D. Roosevelt took office soon after the commission's report was published, his new administration decided health insurance was an issue to be avoided.

The Great Depression would seem to have created the right climate for national health care, but although Roosevelt was personally supportive of the idea, he did not push it. During the depression, medical care did grow as a function of state and local welfare agencies. Many cities and a few states gave beneficiaries a right to needed care at public expense, and welfare agencies provided supplemental payments to help offset medical costs. In 1935 the Resettlement Administration began to set up and subsidize cooperative medical prepayment plans among poor farmers. Under those plans, the local medical societies agreed to accept a limit on the total fees that doctors would receive, essentially creating a form of government-sponsored health insurance.

The depression proved to be a difficult time for the AMA, with many doctors facing unpaid bills and empty waiting rooms. Some local medical associations supported compulsory insurance while others staunchly opposed it. By the mid-1930s the AMA had adjusted its position on voluntary insurance programs, citing those plans that might be acceptable. Most of the AMA members, however, were primarily concerned with operating their practices and were not interested in the political operations of the AMA's leadership.

The only organized dissent to the AMA came from a group of liberal academic physicians called the Committee of Physicians for the Improvement of Medicine. Their statement, signed by over 400 doctors in 1937, called for the formulation of a national health policy, which would include public funding of medical education and research.

In 1937 the Roosevelt administration established the Technical Committee on Medical Care, which was authorized to formulate a national health program. One of the committee's recommendations in its final report was "consideration of a general medical care program supported by taxes, insurance, or both."[3] Roosevelt called a conference in Washington, D.C., to discuss the report, and his reaction to the conference was so enthusiastic that he wanted to make the national health program an issue in the 1938 election.[4]

However, health care never became an issue as a business recession slowed the country again in 1937–38, increasing federal spending and causing many to accuse the New Deal of failure. An epidemic of strikes alarmed businessmen and farmers, and the elections of 1938 produced a conservative backlash. Eighteen states turned against the Democrats, with Republican membership in the House rising from 89 to 170 against 262 Democrats, and in the Senate from 17 to 23 against 69 Democrats.[5] This conservative revival, combined with soon-to-erupt World War II, slowed the momentum for a national health program.

The push for national health insurance began in earnest again during the 1940s. The Wagner-Murray-Dingell bill, introduced in 1943, called for a system of national health insurance as part of a cradle-to-grave social insurance plan. In 1944 Roosevelt asked Congress to affirm an "economic bill of rights," including the right to adequate medical care. President Harry S Truman repeated the request in November 1945, asking Congress to pass a national program to ensure the people's right to medical care. Truman's program was to be a single health insurance system that would cover everyone.

In 1946, however, the Republicans took over Congress. They had their own plans, which emphasized reliance on state and local governments for providing health care for the needy. In 1949, after

[3]Ibid., p. 276.

[4]Ibid., p. 277.

[5]Eugene H. Roseboom, *A History of Presidential Elections* (New York: Macmillan Company, 1957), pp. 458–59.

the election of President Truman, those in Congress and others opposed to national health care mounted a strong campaign linking it to socialized medicine. As anti-communist sentiment rose in the late 1940s and the Truman administration became involved with the Korean War, the prospects for public support for a national health care system vanished. There was little attention to the issue during the more prosperous 1950s.

The 1960s saw a partial adoption of such a system in the Medicare and Medicaid programs and the continued expansion of the Veterans' Administration's medical services. Those programs, which offered treatment to a limited population, were essentially miniversions of a national health care system.

Twenty years after the movement for nationalized health care during the Truman years, Walter Reuther, president of the United Auto Workers, issued a new call for its adoption in a speech to the American Public Health Association in 1968. Reuther helped organize the Committee for National Health Insurance, and in 1969 Sen. Edward Kennedy (D-Mass.), a member of the committee, announced he would introduce legislation. In 1969 the National Governors' Conference (which became the National Governors' Association in the early 1970s) endorsed a plan for national health insurance. By 1970 the AMA, the hospitals, and the insurance industry were all offering their own proposals.

Kennedy's Health Security Plan, introduced in 1970, called for a comprehensive program of free medical care that would replace all public and private health plans with a single, federally operated health insurance system. The plan set a national budget, allocated funds to regions, provided incentives for prepaid group practice, obliged private hospitals and physicians to operate within budget constraints, and required no copayments by patients. Kennedy toured the country holding hearings on his proposal.

In addition to the introduction of Kennedy's plan, in 1970 the Senate Finance Committee approved a social security amendment, introduced by Sen. Russell Long (D-La.), to establish a national insurance program for so-called catastrophic health care costs.

The Nixon administration began preparing an alternative in response to Kennedy's legislation. Out of this planning arose the idea of health maintenance organizations as a method of controlling rising health care costs. By the early 1970s, 26 HMOs were in operation.[6]

In 1974 President Nixon approved a national health insurance plan developed by Health, Education, and Welfare secretary Caspar Weinberger. The plan would have covered the entire population, using private insurance companies to provide coverage for the employed and establishing a separate government-run program for the rest of the population. All patients would pay 25 percent of medical bills, up to a maximum of $1,500 a year. In a message to Congress the president described national health insurance as "an idea whose time has come in America."[7]

During this time, Senator Kennedy offered a bill similar to the president's proposal, but he lost the support of liberals and the unions who wanted his original health security plan. Insurance companies, fearing adoption of the health security plan, urged passage of Senator Long's catastrophic insurance program. Ultimately, Watergate, other political scandals, and the inability of all parties to agree on a specific proposal resulted in stalemate. Again, a national health insurance plan escaped passage.

During the late 1970s both President Jimmy Carter and Senator Kennedy offered competing proposals for national health insurance. The Democrats in Congress had already told the administration that they were not going to consider any plan at that time. Shortly thereafter, Ronald Reagan replaced Carter, and the idea of national health insurance faded from the political landscape.

The 1980s saw further regulation and control of government health programs and the private health care industry, and the explosion in growth of HMOs was spurred by the federal government. Toward the latter part of the decade, with health care costs continuing to spiral, history began to repeat itself as many familiar faces again touted the advantages of a nationalized health care system.

The National Health Care Movement in the 1990s

Not too surprisingly, the AFL-CIO used its national convention in November 1989 to kick off a major campaign for national health insurance legislation. Since then it has spent several million dollars on a campaign aimed at stirring up grass-roots support for national

[6]Starr, p. 396.
[7]Ibid., p. 404.

health insurance, has held hearings in eight cities on the health care issue, and has been offering television programs promoting national health insurance to public broadcasting stations. It is considering whether to support an approach that would impose health-expenditure ceilings or budgets on the government as a whole and on individual states as a way to slow health care spending (similar to the Canadian system) or to accept a plan under which the population would receive federal government-mandated health insurance coverage through employers.[8]

However, what has surprised some (but really shouldn't if one looks at history) are the voices from the business community calling for more federal involvement in health care. Rising health care costs have so frustrated business leaders that some have now resigned themselves to failure and are asking the government to bail them out.

In March 1990 Ford Motor Company, Marriott Corporation, AT&T, E. I. du Pont de Nemours, Eastman Kodak Company, Lockheed Corporation, Minnesota Mining and Manufacturing, Northwest Airlines, and W. R. Grace and Company were among more than a score of U.S. firms that joined with labor to found the National Leadership Coalition for Health Care Reform.[9] Interestingly, in their contract with the Communications Workers of

[8]Unions have been fairly consistent in their support of national health insurance. However, their understanding of the realities under such a system seems cloudy. The kind of health care they would receive under such a program would not be what they expect. According to a 1990 Metropolitan Life survey (conducted by Louis Harris and Associates), which included the responses of 50 union leaders who were overwhelmingly in favor of national health insurance, the union leaders said they believed that "things would get better" with health care under government management (58 percent to 38 percent). However, they had a negative response to limiting the choice of doctors (66 percent to 34 percent), something currently found in HMOs and likely to be included in a national health insurance or mandated-benefits plan. The union leaders were split (50 percent to 50 percent) on whether or not it would be necessary to ration care to control health care costs. The experience with *all* national health care systems has been that rationing becomes an integral part of controlling rising costs when health care budgets are set by the government. Union leaders were also split (50 percent to 50 percent) on the acceptability of waiting several months for elective surgery. Long waits for surgical procedures are well documented for any country with national health care. "Trade-offs & Choices: Health Policy Options for the 1990s," a survey conducted in 1990 for Metropolitan Life Insurance Company by Louis Harris and Associates, New York.

[9]Frank Swoboda, "Major Firms, Unions Join National Health Insurance Bid," *Washington Post*, March 14, 1990, p. F1.

America, AT&T, a member of the coalition, agreed to look for "prompt and lasting national solutions" to rising health care costs.[10]

Art Puccini, a vice president at General Electric, in a speech in 1989, said, "Rising employee medical costs may lead some of us who today are free-market advocates to re-examine our thinking and positions with respect to government-sponsored national health insurance."[11]

Walter B. Maher, director of employee benefits for the Chrysler Corporation, has urged that a national budget be set for health care each year—as is done in Canada, Britain, and other countries with national health care plans. Chrysler estimates that employee health costs add more than $700 to the price of each of its cars. "The cost of health care is eroding standards of living and sapping industrial strength," complained Maher.[12]

The NAM is calling for measures to control rising costs, improve quality, and provide care to as many as 37 million Americans who currently lack health insurance. "I think employers are really going to be the ones to push for major change," said Sharon Conner, an NAM health expert.[13] The NAM has suggested that the Canadian system should be studied. "The Canadian system may not be ideal, but it is food for thought," an NAM official remarked in 1989.[14]

The Washington Business Group on Health, which represents about 180 *Fortune* 500 companies on health issues, is one of several groups drafting a national health care plan (to be released by summer 1992) with the goal of controlling health-related spending.

However, it's not just big business, frustrated with mounting health care costs, that is turning a favorable eye toward a national health plan. A Dun & Bradstreet survey of small businesses found that 38 percent favored some form of national health insurance.[15]

---

[10]Albert R. Karr and Mary Lu Carnevale, "Facing Off over Health-Care Benefits," *Wall Street Journal*, August 11, 1989.

[11]Frank Swoboda and Albert B. Crenshaw, "Pushing for National Health," *Washington Post*, September 3, 1989.

[12]Kenneth H. Bacon, "Business and Labor Reach a Consensus on Need to Reduce Health-Care Costs," *Wall Street Journal*, November 1, 1989.

[13]Ibid.

[14]Swoboda and Crenshaw.

[15]James S. Howard, "Annual Survey: Small Business Presidents Speak Out," *D & B Reports*, November/December 1988, pp. 18–20.

The National Federation of Independent Business says 16 percent of its members polled in 1989 would agree to a mandatory national health insurance program.[16]

In addition to business, some physicians' groups are clamoring for national health care. In 1989 Physicians for a National Health Program, a two-year-old group of 1,200 doctors from across the United States, proposed a single public insurance plan that would pay for all approved medical services. According to Arnold Relman, former editor-in-chief of the *New England Journal of Medicine* and a long-time advocate of a national health care system, "Nothing short of a comprehensive plan is likely to achieve the goals of universal access, cost containment and preservation of quality that everyone seems to want."[17]

The American Academy of Family Physicians released its national health care plan in 1990. It emphasizes mandatory health insurance through use of the private sector and Medicare, as well as a substantially revised and expanded Medicaid program. The AMA is proposing "Health Access America," which would require employers to cover their workers' households, universalize Medicaid for the uncovered poor, create state risk pools for those of modest means who are now "uninsurable," and tax medical fringe benefits.

And finally, the American College of Physicians published a position paper, "Access to Health Care," which concludes that "a comprehensive and coordinated program to [ensure] access on a nationwide basis is essential. New and innovative alternatives will be necessary, including some form of a nationwide financing mechanism to ensure access. To us the times call for a national health policy."[18]

The nation's largest retiree group, the American Association of Retired Persons (AARP), has also jumped on the bandwagon. The AARP is advocating a restructuring of the nation's entire health system to provide comprehensive care for everyone, young and old

[16]Roger Ricklefs, "Health Insurance Becomes a Big Pain for Small Firms," *Wall Street Journal*, December 6, 1989.

[17]Quoted in Glenn Ruffenach, "Physicians' Group Proposes National Health Program," *Wall Street Journal*, November 12, 1989.

[18]American College of Physicians, "Universal Access to Health Care in America: A Moral and Medical Imperative," *Annals of Internal Medicine* 112, no. 9 (May 1, 1990).

alike. Interestingly, AARP officials say it was the defeat by the elderly of the catastrophic insurance program in 1989 that persuaded it to adopt the new cause. That organization believes it would be easier to overhaul the entire system than to win new benefits for the elderly alone. "The status quo isn't acceptable," said Horace Deets, AARP's executive director. "We need something that's universal, that's perceived as equitable and that's shared by everybody. It's got to be from cradle to grave."[19]

Some recent polling seems to show that even segments of the general population are looking to the federal government to solve the nation's health care problems. In a June 1991 poll by the *Wall Street Journal* and NBC News, 51 percent of 1,006 registered voters said that the federal government had primary responsibility for solving the problem of the high cost of health care.[20] By 69 percent to 28 percent, voters supported the idea of guaranteeing everyone the "best" health care available even if it takes a tax increase to pay for it; in addition, 69 percent supported the adoption of a Canadian-style system, while 20 percent were opposed.[21]

However, 70 percent of those interviewed in the *Wall Street Journal*/NBC News poll felt that everyone should be required to pay some share of medical expenses. Obviously, the general public does not understand just what is at stake in a national health care plan; those interviewed agreed (by a margin of 52 percent to 42 percent) that they were unwilling to limit the types of tests and procedures available under insurance and government programs.[22] Such limitations have been imposed under every nationalized health care plan now in existence, and they would be imposed under any plan the United States would adopt.

Our brief look at history shows that the seemingly unusual coalition of groups supporting nationalized health care is not new; indeed, it has existed in various forms off and on throughout the 20th century. Some of the organizations currently promoting

---

[19]Kenneth H. Bacon, "AARP, Now Championing Health Care for All, Scrambles to Prove It's More Than a Paper Tiger," *Wall Street Journal*, December 27, 1989.

[20]Michel McQueen, "Voters, Sick of the Current Health-Care System, Want Federal Government to Prescribe Remedy," *Wall Street Journal*, June 28, 1991. Fifty-five percent said the "high cost of health care" was the most important issue.

[21]Ibid.

[22]Ibid.

nationalized care are drawing on the examples of Canada, Britain, and other countries for their proposals, and others are pushing a mandated-benefits approach such as those found in Massachusetts, Hawaii, and a few other states.

Next, the various programs will be examined, their strengths and weaknesses will be noted, and conclusions will be drawn about their success in providing universal, high-quality care while controlling health care costs.

Health Care Systems in Other Countries

In most countries, government plays a much greater role in financing and operating health care systems than the U.S. government does.[23] These systems encompass a wide variety of government-run programs; many use the private market to some degree.

The British System

The British National Health Service was created in 1948 as the free world's first comprehensive government health care system. The system provides cradle-to-grave health services for British citizens. Britons have access to a general practitioner—although not usually one of their choosing—at no charge and can obtain prescription drugs at a nominal cost of less than $4, although 80 percent of the population is exempt from even that charge.

There are no hospital or physician charges for tests or in-hospital treatment. The system is financed primarily through general tax revenues, and the proceeds divided among regional health authorities that plan local health services. The regions split their cash among districts that pay for hospitals through global prospective budgets. A very small contribution is made through payroll taxes and by private patients who pay fees for the use of hospital facilities under the supervision of their own private physician. About a tenth of Britons have private insurance.

The national government owns and operates over 2,000 hospitals and directly employs most hospital staff, although some hospital physicians, like most general practitioners and dentists, combine their work with private practice. With about 1 million employees,

---

[23]This account of the structure of foreign health care systems is taken from Stuart M. Butler and Edmund F. Haislmaier, eds., *Critical Issues: A National Health System for America* (Washington: Heritage Foundation, 1989), pp. 38–40.

including over 50,000 physicians, the National Health Service is one of the world's largest employers.

The Swedish System

Sweden provides a universal government health care system, run mainly by local county councils. The councils own Sweden's public-sector hospitals and, as a group, negotiate salaries with physicians, nurses, and ancillary workers. About 5 percent of the physicians are in private practice, mainly in the cities, and they account for about 20 percent of ambulatory medical care.

Nearly all the financing for the Swedish system comes from payroll taxes or general taxes. Patient charges, however, are high compared to those in most European countries. There is a charge of approximately $8.50 for each of the first 15 visits to a doctor, a $10 charge for drugs, and a daily hospital fee of $8.50. Despite a national population that is only one-seventh that of Britain, the Swedish health system employs about one-third as many workers as does the British system.

The German System

The German health system is a refinement of a compulsory social insurance system first developed in 1883 by Chancellor Otto von Bismarck. It is the world's oldest social insurance system. All Germans other than a few who are privately insured are enrolled in the system. Matching contributions from employers and employees are channeled to about 1,400 so-called sickness funds, or nonprofit insurance companies, to which Germans must belong. Each sickness fund sets it own rate, which is collected as a tax on earnings up to a certain annually adjusted level, known as the wage base. The average tax rate is 13 percent, split between the employer and the employee. Dependents are automatically enrolled, and the unemployed also are enrolled, with premiums paid on their behalf by the government. Patients are not charged for visits to a physician, but they do pay just over $1 for prescriptions and just over $3 per day for a hospital stay.

Hospitals and physicians must negotiate fees with the sickness funds. General practitioners and other office-based physicians are grouped in regional associations of insurance doctors. In exchange for agreed-upon services, based on a minimum established by law, each sickness fund pays the regional association a certain amount, and the association distributes this money according to a fee schedule agreed upon by the association members. Patients have free choice among the physicians who agree to treat sickness fund patients—and those physicians represent about 90 percent of general practitioners.

Payments to hospitals take two forms. The German federal government regulates the daily charges that hospitals can bill the sickness funds for treating patients. In addition, federal, state, and local authorities reimburse hospitals for the cost of construction and equipment.

The Dutch System

The Netherlands, like Germany, has a social insurance system run by sickness funds. The system has three main components: catastrophic insurance for everybody, run by the government; a social insurance system for the bottom two-thirds of earners; and private insurance for the rest. Most Dutch providers are private hospitals and fee-for-service doctors, although there is a patchy arrangement of general practitioners who are paid according to the number of patients they treat. Since 1983 hospitals have been paid out of global prospective budgets.

A Critique of the British, Swedish, German, and Dutch Health Care Systems

One point in favor of the national health care plans in other countries is that they appear to be very popular with voters. A poll in Britain in June 1988 found 64 percent of Britons rating the National Health Service as "good" and only 15 percent rating it as "poor."[24] The poll also found that 64 percent favored "total state (central government)" funding for the service, in contrast to only 2 percent who favored "mainly or solely" private funding for health.[25]

In spite of the strong popular support for such national health care systems, there is criticism among the patients. Most assume that the problems they encounter are attributable to a lack of government funding, however, not to flaws inherent in the system.

---

[24]Poll conducted in June 1988 by Market & Opinion Research International Ltd., as reported in Steve Lohr, "For Britain's Health Service, Little Cash but Big Demands," *New York Times*, August 7, 1988.

[25]Ibid.

The champions of foreign health care programs point to certain statistics, usually infant mortality rates, to support their argument that such systems lead to improved health for the general population. But comparing the effectiveness of health care systems is not as straightforward as it may seem. According to Uwe Reinhardt of Princeton University:

> These crude indicators tell us little about the relative efficacy of different health systems, because these health-status indicators are shaped by many socioeconomic and demographic factors completely outside the control of the health system proper. It would therefore be neither meaningful nor fair to read into such crude numbers shortcomings of the American health system per se.[26]

The root cause of problems within foreign national health care systems is the same problem that contributes to rising health care costs in the United States: patients contribute little or nothing to the cost of their care. This little-or-no deductible or copayment policy leads to increased demand for services, resulting in spiraling costs and out-of-control government budgets and private-market costs. In countries with national health care budgets determined by the political process, the increasing demand for services outgrows the supply of government funds, resulting in chronic shortages, deficiencies, and rationing of medical services and supplies.

Despite a budget increase in real terms of nearly one-third since Margaret Thatcher became prime minister in 1979, the National Health Service's $38.7 billion-a-year program is in chaos. Over 1 million citizens are on the waiting list for elective surgery.[27] Government figures indicate that 25 percent of those on the list will be kept waiting for more than a year.[28] Men over the age of 55 cannot normally get kidney dialysis. Richard Clarke, an American consultant to the service, noted that while Britain spends much less on health care than the United States does (6.1 percent of GNP versus

---

[26]Uwe E. Reinhardt, "Health Care Expenditures in Other Countries," statement presented to the Subcommittee on Education and Health, Joint Economic Committee of the U.S. Congress, May 3, 1987.

[27]"Health Care: Survey," *Economist*, July 6, 1991, p. 12.

[28]Butler and Haislmaier, p. 45.

11 percent), the care is rendered in a state of "startling inefficiency."[29] For example, by working longer hours, an American
orthopedist might do twice as many hip replacements as his salaried
British counterpart.[30] Government controls have led to serious complaints by medical personnel about pay, to high rates of emigration
by physicians, and to strikes by other medical personnel. Britain
has one of the lowest rates of physicians per unit of population of
any Western industrialized country.[31]

Price controls, rationing, and waiting lists do put a lid on health
care spending, and that is why many politicians can boast that
countries with national health care programs seem to spend less on
health care than does the United States.

Government spending priorities affect other areas of health care.
For example, Goran Lennmaker, a health care expert, pointed out
that chronic hospital bed shortages in Sweden are attributable to
the fact that "government has monopolized health care."[32]

Rationing the use of high-technology equipment is common in
all countries with national health care systems; long waits for specific tests and treatments are commonplace. In Sweden a recent
government commission on coronary care found that Swedes can
wait up to 11 months for a diagnostic heart X-ray, and up to 8
months more for essential heart surgery. A research cardiologist
calculated that at least 1,000 Swedes die each year for lack of heart
treatment.[33]

The German government limits the number of training slots allot-
ted to specialists. Dr. Isabelle Richmond, a neurosurgeon who
worked for the U.S. Army in the 1980s, examined dozens of soldiers
and dependents who suffered brain tumors, head wounds, and
other serious injuries while stationed in Germany. Because that
country has relatively few neurosurgeons, some of the victims were
operated on by general surgeons. Richmond remarked, "Patients

[29]Association of American Physicians and Surgeons, "A National Health Plan: Rx
for Bankruptcy," *AAPS News* 46, no. 7 (July 1990), p. 1.

[30]Ibid.

[31]Butler and Haislmaier, p. 44.

[32]Quoted in Annika Schildt, "In Sweden, Equality Is Tinged with Inefficiency,"
Washington Post, August 16, 1988.

[33]Ibid.

who in the U.S. would have been restored to functioning people were left as gorks."[34]

Several of the European governments, battling budget problems and escalating health care costs, have introduced some market-oriented reforms into their systems. The Dutch government is grappling with a package of pro-competitive reforms that would encourage regulated competition among insurers, who would buy selectively from competing health care providers. The Germans are struggling with a string of cost-containment laws. Swedish county councils are revamping their monolithic health care system to create competition and more patient choice. Other European countries—including Ireland and Denmark—are pushing for more competition in health care to improve efficiency. Within the European Community, a market in cross-border health care, sometimes known as medical tourism, is emerging. Patients fed up with waiting or bad care go elsewhere and charge the cost to their homeland.

The Canadian System

> TORONTO—Stella Lacroix's death started as a suicide. But most people here think it ended as something else. Moments after she swallowed a quart of cleaning fluid, she changed her mind and raced to the nearest emergency room. The hospital wasn't equipped to perform the surgery she needed to stop internal bleeding, so her doctor began a frantic search for an available bed elsewhere in the Toronto area.
>
> "She was turned away from 14 hospitals," the doctor, Derek Nesdoly, said after his three-hour search had failed. "There was no space anywhere and she just bled to death. This woman needed immediate care and we couldn't get it for her." The death caused outrage in Canada, where the government guarantees its citizens universal access to competent health care at no charge.[35]

Since 1971 all of Canada's provinces have provided universal hospital and physician insurance. The federal government contributes approximately 50 percent of the cost (more in the poorer provinces), and the provinces are responsible for the rest. Health

[34]Lee Smith, "A Cure for What Ails Medical Care," *Fortune*, July 1, 1991, p. 44.

[35]Michael Specter, "Health Care in Canada: A Model with Limits," *Washington Post*, December 18, 1989.

care funding is channeled through provincial health care programs that in some cases are administered by single corporations. Canadians have free choice of hospitals and doctors and pay virtually nothing directly. Most Canadians are covered by some form of supplemental insurance that pays for additional services not covered under the provincial plans. Supplemental insurance is often provided by employers as an employee benefit.

In some provinces a mixture of income and sales taxes pays for the provincial portion, but in Alberta and Ontario the system is based on social insurance principles, and residents are required to pay premiums, usually deducted from payroll checks. In Ontario about 70 percent of the population pays premiums directly or indirectly through their employers. Residents over the age of 65 receive services without paying premiums, as do individuals and families without sufficient resources. Total premiums contribute about 20 percent of the health insurance budget.

The vast majority of hospital beds in Canada are in private institutions. The insurance program in each province reimburses hospitals on the basis of their operating costs. A calculation is made of the likely utilization rate in the area, and the acceptable total cost of services is determined by a rate-setting body in each province. This body is usually appointed by the minister of health, who gives a major role in the body's membership selection to the insurance plan. Hospitals are permitted to charge fees for special services directly to patients. The capital expenditures of hospitals are financed by government grants, or the money is raised privately.

Fee for service is the dominant form of payment to physicians, for both hospital and office services, although some hospital doctors are paid a salary (but fees are fixed). All physicians are reimbursed according to a fee schedule for services, which is negotiated with the provincial medical associations.

A Critique of the Canadian Health Care System

As in Britain, there is strong support for the public health system in Canada, as reflected in a 1988 poll in which 81 percent of respondents declared they were "very" or "quite" satisfied with the plan.[36] However, the system has not been in place as long as the other foreign systems, and the difficulties that already abound in those

[36]Lohr.

systems are beginning to appear within the Canadian system. Stories of dissatisfaction and disaster are on the increase—witness the story of Stella Lacroix.

New technology is less available to patients in Canada than to those in the United States. For example, the United States has 2,000 magnetic resonance imaging machines, whereas Canada has only 15.[37] Provincial governments control the introduction of technology. A hospital can raise private funds to purchase such a machine, but because the money to continue its operation comes from the government and the government won't always authorize such funds, hospitals cannot afford to buy the equipment they need. Furthermore, doctors can't bill the government for use of the equipment unless it is authorized. Consequently, new technology has been introduced more slowly than in the United States. For example, the entire province of Newfoundland, with a population of 579,000, has a single CAT scanner, compared to the city of Tucson, Arizona, which is similar in size and has 11.[38] The city of Seattle, Washington, population 500,000, has more CAT scanners than the province of British Columbia, population 3 million.[39]

The slower implementation of technology means waiting lists for some procedures. Government controls the type and frequency of many diagnostic tests. A person suspected of having a brain tumor doesn't immediately receive a CAT scan and may have to wait several weeks for one. In Newfoundland an "urgent" pap smear, used to detect cervical cancer, routinely takes two months.[40] Many experts agree that Canada has held its costs down in part by limiting the number of certain procedures such as coronary bypasses and angiograms. In Ottawa a heart patient can expect to wait four months for a coronary bypass operation.[41] In Toronto the wait can be up to a year.[42] According to one account:

[37] Smith, "A Cure for What Ails Medical Care."

[38] Data on Newfoundland are from Michael A. Walker, "Neighborly Advice on Health Care," *Wall Street Journal*, June 8, 1988; data on Tucson based on personal communication from Daniel Anavy, Nuclear Medicine Department, St. Joseph's Hospital, Tucson.

[39] Don Feder, "The High Cost of National Health Insurance," *Human Events*, June 15, 1991.

[40] Ibid.

[41] Michael Malloy, "Health, Canadian Style," *Wall Street Journal*, April 22, 1988.

[42] Feder.

Malcolm Stevens of British Columbia needed a coronary bypass, but because of the waiting list for this procedure, he was told that he would have to wait six months to a year. Two months after his diagnosis, on July 10, 1982, he died of a heart attack. Ironically, the same day, his doctor bumped another patient from the schedule to make room for Stevens.[43]

According to the AMA, Canada has only 11 heart surgery facilities, one for every 2.3 million residents. In the United States there are 793 such facilities, one for every 300,000 people. Long waiting lists for medical care would seem to negate the ideal of national health care (that everyone receive high-quality care) and they represent an inferior method of keeping down demand.[44]

A shortage of hospital beds in Canada is becoming the norm. In efforts to control health care spending, which in Ontario rose from 26 percent of the provincial budget in 1978 to more than one-third in 1989, hospital spending has been curtailed.[45] That cutback has led to occasional shortages of beds, and in September 1989 it caused officials of Toronto's Princess Margaret Hospital, one of the nation's best cancer facilities, to announce that they would take no new patients for six weeks.[46] In Brampton, Ontario, Thomas Dickson, head of surgery at Peel Memorial Hospital, said, "We don't have enough beds. We sometimes have to cancel surgery for lack of beds."[47]

---

[43]The House Wednesday Group, Congress of the United States, *Public Health in the Provinces: Canadian National Health Insurance Strategy* (Washington, 1989), p. 14.

[44]In 1990 the Fraser Institute in Vancouver, British Columbia, published the first comprehensive scientific survey of waiting lists in the Canadian health system. The average waiting time for the 20 least available treatments in British Columbia ranged from 6 weeks for a D & C to 33 weeks for septal surgery. A child's tonsillectomy requires a wait of 14 weeks, and a hysterectomy is delayed for 16 weeks. Some 522 children are waiting for a tonsillectomy, and 206 women are waiting for a hysterectomy. Additional information on various procedures and waiting periods can be found in Steven Globerman and Lorna Hoye, "Waiting Your Turn: Hospital Waiting Lists in Canada," *Critical Issues Bulletin* (Vancouver, B.C.: Fraser Institute, May 1990).

[45]Specter.

[46]Ibid.

[47]Malloy.

WHAT HAS GOVERNMENT DONE TO OUR HEALTH CARE?

Sometimes the shortage of hospital beds has resulted in calamities worse than the inconvenience of a postponed surgery. On some occasions it has resulted in a patient's death, as was the case of little Joel Bondy.

> Two-year-old Joel Bondy was slated for cardiac surgery in January 1990 in London, Ontario. His operation was repeatedly postponed, as more critical cases were moved up. Alarmed at their son's deteriorating condition, Joel's parents got in touch with Heartbeat Windsor, a private, voluntary organization founded in 1989 that helps Canadians obtain critically needed surgery in the U.S. Heartbeat Windsor got Joel scheduled for surgery in Detroit. Ontario officials, embarrassed by media coverage of Joel's condition, informed the family that Joel could have his operation immediately—in Toronto. After a four-hour ambulance ride, a hospital bed was not available. The family had to spend the night in a hotel, and Joel Bondy died the next day, four hours before his surgery.[48]

The lack of technology, coupled with rationing and shortages, results in inadequate care, not the "quality care" the Canadian system is supposed to deliver. For example, consider the American woman who suffered a heart attack while visiting a son in Canada.[49] Conveniently, all medical costs were covered by Canada's socialized medicine. However, the family questions the quality of her care because the Canadian physicians would not reveal their treatment methods. Furthermore, all the doctors involved have refused to forward any of her records to the United States. This left her personal physician back home in a quandary as to the treatment he should prescribe because he did not know any details of her heart attack or treatment.

In a similar case, Michael Billett, founder and operator of Heartbeat Windsor, reported that Canadian doctors refused to dispatch Monique Nadon's medical records to Cleveland, where her heart surgery was scheduled. "There were about 2½ weeks of angry phone calls, threats of legal action and a lot of lies about 'shipping

---

[48]John A. Barnes, "Canadians Cross Border to Save Their Lives," *Wall Street Journal*, December 12, 1990.

[49]From an interview with the author.

problems,' " said Monique's father, Patrick Nadon. Monique finally had her surgery, however, and recovered.[50]

The Canadian government boasts that no one who is ill is denied prompt medical care. If patients need emergency care and the local hospital has no facilities or equipment to provide it, they are transported to the nearest hospital that does. If necessary services are available only in another province, or in the United States, the patient goes there. In the cases of Stella Lacroix, Joel Bondy, Monique Nadon, and Malcolm Stevens, however, this system of "prompt and quality care" failed miserably.

Canada also has experimented with additional controls on its ever-increasing costs. Some critics believe that the politicians, rather than risk voter backlash by raising taxes, are threatening quality of care even further with other controls on spending. In Quebec, for example, there are caps on doctors' incomes. When a general practitioner's gross quarterly income (before taxes and overhead) reaches the U.S. equivalent of $37,102, the government will pay him or her only 25 percent of the usual fee for the rest of the quarter.[51] This restriction, in effect, caps a doctor's income at approximately $148,000 a year, which must certainly affect productivity and quality of care. "The increasing government control of what we can earn is very frustrating. If I see a patient with the flu in my office, I can't charge more than $20," said Michael Wyman, a Toronto physician in family practice.[52]

Ontario physicians are allowed to bill for only two hours of endometriosis surgery. Even if they are willing to work without payment after that, there is the problem of getting the operating room and other staff for the seven hours that might be needed. The solution: a network for referring patients to physicians in Bend, Oregon.[53]

Many Canadian physicians are angry about the fee restrictions imposed on them and also about other controls they believe interfere with the practice of medicine. Until 1984 some provinces allowed physicians to "balance bill" patients above the agreed fee

[50]Barnes.

[51]"The Crisis in Health Insurance: A Look at the Canadian Alternative," *Consumer Reports*, September 1990, p. 614.

[52]Specter.

[53]*Today's Health*, December 1990.

schedule. But a federal law cut federal assistance to provinces that permitted extra billings. The action was fought by some physicians, and in Ontario it triggered a 25-day strike by doctors.

The British Columbia government recently decided to restrict, by region and specialty, the number of new physicians entitled to get insurance payments. This action amounts to dictating where a new doctor can practice by refusing to provide "billing numbers" to new practitioners. "They are very frustrated, very upset, very mad," Janet Martini said of young physicians in the province. With a few months remaining in her residency in geriatric medicine, she still didn't know if the province would let her take a hospital appointment she had planned on for the past three years.[54] The Quebec government, by preferential or punitive payment practice, forces newly practicing doctors to provide services where it chooses.

According to Dr. William Goodman, a specialist in Toronto who has been on strike since 1986:

> The bureaucratic establishment of mandatory norms for doctors and hospitals is rapidly leading to a government-directed, assembly-line, civil-service type of practice. Computers run by nonmedical, politically appointed medical administrators are progressively replacing medical judgment. Canadian medical bureaucrats now make the decisions on what care shall be made available, not individual patients in concert with their personal physicians.[55]

Some physicians, fed up with the system, have either quit the practice of medicine or immigrated to the United States. As Goodman remarked, "The emigration or early retirement of many of our best physicians [has] left large gaps in the medical, hospital, and university hierarchies."[56]

The answer for many patients, frustrated by the lack of available treatment, has been the same—go to the United States. Interestingly, even though Canadians cannot buy private insurance coverage for health care in their own country, they are allowed to buy policies to cover care in the United States. Because 90 percent of

[54]Malloy.

[55]William E. Goodman, "Canadian Medicare: A Road to Serfdom," Association of American Physicians and Surgeons, pamphlet no. 1012, August 1990, pp. 9, 11.

[56]Ibid., p. 9.

Canadians live within 100 miles of the U.S. border, it's no problem for them to drive to a dozen or more major American cities. This option allows them an escape route from the rationing and waiting lines in their homeland. The magazine *Hospitals* reported that in the first five months of 1989, half of the patients receiving lithotripsy, a technique used to treat kidney stones, at Buffalo General Hospital were Canadians.[57] Michael Billett, who founded Heartbeat Windsor after he was forced to go to the United States for his own heart surgery, said his organization helped 600 patients get to the United States for surgery in 1990.[58] And at the Cleveland Clinic, approximately 100 Canadians undergo heart surgery every year.[59]

This kind of government control creates a two-tiered system of health care because only those who can afford the expense of traveling to the United States can take advantage of the more available care. As Canadians watch the health care debate in the United States, they must wonder, If the United States adopts a health care system similar to ours, what will happen to our safety net?

Has the Canadian System Controlled Health Care Costs?

Proponents of nationalized health care systems, using data that compare the health care spending of the two countries relative to their gross national products, claim that Canada spends much less than the United States on health care. In 1967 both countries spent relatively the same amount of GNP on health care, approximately 6 percent. By 1971, when the main components of Canada's national health care system were in place, both countries were spending a little above 7 percent. In the years following, the rates of growth compared to GNP began to diverge, with Canada spending less of its GNP on health care; by 1987 Canada's national health expenditures as a share of GNP were 9 percent, compared to the U.S. share at 11 percent.[60]

---

[57]Stuart A. Wesbury, Jr., "Doctors after Hours," *Washington Post*, March 18, 1990, p. B3.

[58]John C. Goodman, "Wrong Prescription for the Uninsured," *Wall Street Journal*, June 11, 1991.

[59]Ibid.

[60]Edward Neuschler, *Canadian Health Care: The Implications of Public Health Insurance* (Washington: Health Insurance Association of America, June 1990).

However, comparing the health care spending of the two countries solely on the basis of GNP is misleading and inaccurate. In many countries, such as Canada and Japan, the level of health care spending as a percentage of GNP can appear low by international standards. But success in attaining cost control in health care spending is a reflection not of a better system but of faster GNP growth.

Edward Neuschler of the Health Insurance Association of America conducted a study that compared health care spending in Canada and the United States for the period 1967–87.[61]Neuschler adjusted the figures to eliminate distortions caused by differences in economic growth rates (GNP), which were higher in Canada than in the United States during this period. To eliminate this distortion and others, including differences in inflation rates, population growth rates, and currency exchange rates, he calculated health care spending for both countries on a per capita basis in constant dollars in each country's own currency. The results showed almost parallel rates of increase in health spending for both Canada and the United States.[62]

Neuschler also corrected for baseline differences in spending levels in 1967, thereby making it possible to compare expenditure growth with the same baseline amount in each country.[63]Consequently, he was able to determine that the cumulative growth in real per capita spending for both countries was almost identical.[64]

Advocates of the Canadian system claim that one of the main reasons Canada has achieved lower health care costs than the United States is that its system is more efficient and has lower administrative costs due to a centralized bureaucracy. They assert

[61]Ibid.

[62]U.S. per capita health care spending rose from approximately $700 in 1967 to approximately $1,600 in 1987. In Canada the rate rose from approximately $600 in 1967 to $1,500 in 1987. See Neuschler.

[63]Neuschler corrected for baseline differences by calculating each country's real per capita health spending as the ratio of spending in each year to spending in 1967.

[64]Starting with a baseline of 1 percent for both countries, the cumulative increase since 1967 in real health care spending per capita for the United States rose to approximately 2.5 percent, a little below the increase for Canada, which was also approximately 2.5 percent. Another study examining the real differences in spending growth between the United States and Canada is Jacques Krasny and Ian R. Ferrier, *The Canadian Healthcare System in Perspective* (Morristown, N.J.: Borgart Delafield Ferrier, July 1990).

that government monopolies can reduce overhead costs by economies of scale and do not incur the marketing costs found in the U.S. system. However, students of economics know that, in the long run, all monopolies become increasingly inefficient when there is lack of pressure to compete and, as a result, extremely costly to operate. Even so, when accurate cost comparisons are made, as they are in the Neuschler study, the supposed savings attributed to the Canadian system vanish, making any efficiency arguments invalid. In addition, the costs incurred in having the bureaucracy collect and redistribute the tax monies for health care are not included in cost estimates of the Canadian system.

In 1991 there were reports from Canada that, owing to cuts in the federal budget, a bill passed in 1990 (Bill C–69) would substantially cut and eventually eliminate the federal contribution to health care. It would gradually bring to an end the transfer payments from Ottawa to the provincial health plans, thereby causing the death of the Canadian national health plan as early as 1994. According to Dr. Harry Watts, chairman of the Newfoundland Medical Association, "The federal government has found itself trying to cope with a large deficit and interest payments. In one swift, deft legislative manoeuvre the federal government has signalled that it is getting out of the health care business."[65] When the federal government no longer transfers cash, it will lose the ability to enforce the Canada Health Act, and provinces will be free to institute private insurance and extra billing. Dr. Michael Rachlis, Toronto Board of Health, commented that "without control over spending, the federal government would be unable to prevent some provinces from going to a totally American system."[66]

Watts admitted that the federal spending cuts will come at a time when "health care costs are rising above the rate of inflation" (so much for the cost-control pluses of a national health care plan) and that the passage of C–69 means that "the federal government loses the moral and fiscal 'big stick' to hold over provinces."[67] However, he also admitted that the demise of the national health care system

[65]Jane Coutts, "Medicare May Soon Be Dead, Report Says," *Toronto Globe and Mail*, June 7, 1991, p. A10.
[66]Harry Watts, "Bill C-69: An End to Universality?" *Family Practice*, April 6, 1991.
[67]Ibid.

may have some pluses. "The provinces may be able to introduce alternate payment mechanisms which may promote *greater individual responsibility* for health and reduce the burden on the system."[68]

Would a Canadian-Style System Work in the United States?

Stuart A. Wesbury, Jr., president of the American College of Healthcare Executives, has written that "the United States is not prepared to accept nationalized health care, nor is there any alternative system that can realistically be substituted for our own."[69] In his view, although the United States does have problems with its health care system, the solutions must be tailored to the needs of American society, not based on a foreign model. Different cultures have different requirements, desires, and expectations, and Wesbury says that proponents of nationalized health care too often ignore these differences.

According to John B. Crosby, senior vice president of health policy development for the AMA:

> America's political culture and general cultural values are critical factors in determining public policy. Present and future U.S. health policies are usually anchored in the past. . . . Americans may not be like Canadians, Germans and others in accepting and using the health-care system, and may also have a different outlook on the role of government in social policy. This isn't to say we can't learn from the experiences of other countries, but a look around the world provides no ready-made answer to how America's system should be modified.[70]

Wesbury cited several reasons why he believes a Canadian-style system would not work in the United States. One is that the high U.S. standard of living demands a higher quality of health care, something that nationalized systems have difficulty reaching and maintaining. Another reason is patient expectation. Americans are not inclined to wait in line for care, as many in other countries do. Most Americans would find delays for surgery and other treatment unacceptable. A third reason is our dependence on technology.

[68]Ibid. Emphasis added.

[69]Stuart A. Wesbury, Jr., "Why Other Nations' Rx Won't Work," *Washington Post*, March 18, 1990, p. B3.

[70]John B. Crosby, letter to the editor, *Wall Street Journal*, July 17, 1991.

According to Wesbury, the U.S. consumer demands the latest in diagnostic and therapeutic hardware before economies of scale or competition can bring the price down. Such technology has prolonged life, reduced inpatient admissions and length of stay, and dramatically improved the practice of medicine. It has also increased the cost.

A fourth reason, according to Wesbury, involves ethical issues. Americans are not predisposed to ration or restrict care to certain people, such as impaired or premature newborns and the elderly. Swedish doctors withhold any treatment from infants with a grim prognosis; in the Netherlands, gravely ill patients are given the option of euthanasia; and Britain rations such services as kidney dialysis and hip replacements for patients above certain ages.[71]

The issue of physicians' quitting or taking early retirement would surely arise in the United States following implementation of a Canadian-style program. Many physicians would not like such a system, and more than a few might discontinue practicing if such a program were enacted.

What Would a Canadian-Style System Cost the United States?

According to three recent studies, the costs of adopting a Canadian-style system would range from $12 billion to as much as $339 billion a year.

The Neuschler study calculated that the United States would need an additonal $189 billion a year in spending to finance a Canadian-style system.[72] Neuschler stated that 74 percent of Canadian health spending is funded by the public sector, whereas only 42 percent of U.S. spending is public.[73] Raising U.S. public-sector funding to 74 percent (in 1988) would have required an additional $179 billion a year, and expanding coverage to the uninsured would have required $10 billion a year, for a total of $189 billion.[74]

A study released by the National Center for Policy Analysis, a Dallas-based research institute, stated that adopting a Canadian-style national health insurance program would require $339 billion

---

[71]Wesbury, "Why Other Nations' Rx Won't Work."
[72]Neuschler.
[73]Ibid.
[74]Ibid.

in additional taxes, increasing the U.S. budget by almost one-third.[75] Gary Robbins, an economist who coauthored the study, said, "The government would have to increase income tax rates by 14 percentage points, or increase the payroll tax rate by 15 percentage points, or enact a value-added tax equal to almost 10 percent of the value of all goods and services."[76]

The study concluded that many U.S. employers would find that the costs of paying for such a system would be higher than their current health care costs, and that large manufacturing companies would be hit hardest, hurting America's international competitiveness. High-wage industries, such as the automobile industry, would pay above-average taxes, even though their workers would receive the same benefits as other workers. For example, the automobile industry would pay about $5,641 per employee per year under a national health insurance payroll tax. Add the loss of the current deduction for private health insurance and the total cost rises to $6,824 per worker per year. Because the automobile industry now pays only $3,055 for private health insurance, the cost of health care for auto workers would more than double under national health insurance.

The adoption of a Canadian-style program in the United States would result in widespread income redistribution among industries, with low-wage industries benefiting over high-wage industries. Those industries with below-average wages would pay below-average national health insurance rates. That would put them at a financial and competitive advantage over some of the high-wage industries that are now calling for a national health care program.

PNHP Proposal for Nationalized Health Care

Physicians for a National Health Care Program (PNHP) has proposed a national health care plan. In drawing heavily from the Canadian program, however, PNHP is recommending that the United States adopt a system that is increasingly troublesome for both the government and the people of Canada.

---

[75]Gary Robbins and Aldona Robbins, *What a Canadian-Style Health Care System Would Cost U.S. Employers and Employees*, NCPA Policy Report no. 145 (Dallas: National Center for Policy Analysis, February 1990).

[76]Press release accompanying ibid.

According to cost estimates provided for PNHP by Lewin/ICF, an additional $12.2 billion per year in total health care spending over 1991 spending levels would be required to make the utilization of health care by the uninsured commensurate with its use by the insured.[77] PNHP also expects savings of $31 billion in hospital administrative costs and $9 billion in physician administrative costs as a result of reduced paperwork. According to PNHP, if the system operated with the administrative efficiency of the Canadian system,[78] these savings would result in a total health care cost savings of $55 billion over the 1991 estimates of $602 billion.[79]

PNHP recommends that neither copayments nor deductibles be paid by patients. It claims that Canada has few such charges, yet health costs are lower than in the United States and have risen slowly. However, copayments and deductibles have little to do with any supposedly lower health care costs in Canada. Lower costs, if there are any, are attributable to rationing and the controls placed on service by the federal government. The lack of copayments and deductibles actually serves to increase demand and raise costs, as any first-year economics student learns. Even PNHP admits, "We are uncertain how utilization patterns might respond to universal, first-dollar insurance coverage."[80]

PNHP recommends centralized, bureaucratic control of technology, services covered, capital allocations, and prescription drugs. In Canada, such centralized control has resulted in a lack of available technology, rationing of care, and excessive control of physicians' practices, which have contributed to doctors' taking early retirement and immigrating to the United States. Centralized planning of coverage and benefits also prevents the development of variations that better meet local and individual needs.

PNHP recommends centralized control of hospital capital expenditures to facilitate "rational planning." The Canadian government claims that it has been successful in containing costs and improving

---

[77]Kevin Grumbach et al., "Liberal Benefits, Conservative Spending," *Journal of the American Medical Association* 265, no. 19 (May 15, 1991).

[78]Grounds for skepticism about the efficiency of the Canadian system were discussed earlier in relation to the Neuschler study.

[79]Grumbach et al.

[80]Ibid., p. 2551.

the distribution of health resources. But according to William Goodman, centralized control of hospitals in Canada has contributed to "chronic understaffing as well as an inability of hospitals to provide the high-tech expensive machinery needed for state-of-the-art diagnosis and treatment."[81] And, as mentioned earlier, costs are out of control.

PNHP claims that, as in the Canadian system, U.S. physicians would see less bureaucratic interference in clinical decisionmaking. In Canada, however, greater government involvement in the practice of medicine, with controls on volume, utilization, costs, and quality reviews, has resulted in further losses of physician autonomy. Government decisions to ration care directly limit medical decisionmaking.

According to PNHP, employers that now provide generous employee benefits would realize a saving because their contribution to the program would be less than their current health care costs. However, as shown in the Robbins and Robbins study for NCPA, many companies, particularly those in high-wage industries that already offer generous employee benefits, would find their health care burden higher under a PNHP-type program. The Robbinses concluded that payroll taxes would have to increase to cover the $339 billion in new revenues that they estimate would be necessary to fund such a program.[82] PNHP emphasizes that "the average individual and business would not pay more for health care under the PNHP but would pay taxes that take the place of, but do not exceed, current premium payments and out-of-pocket costs."[83] Funding for the PNHP's new program would come approximately 38 percent from payroll taxes; 26 percent from federal, state, and local revenues; and 21 percent from new federal tax revenues.[84]

PNHP concludes that overall health costs would rise less steeply because of improved health planning and greater efficiency. However, that has not been the case in Canada. As William Goodman has stated, "It took almost 20 years after the introduction of socialized medicine in Ontario for the politicians to grudgingly acknowledge, as our Minister of Health did last year, that 'health care

[81]Goodman, "Canadian Medicare," p. 3.

[82]Robbins and Robbins.

[83]Quoted in Grumbach et al., p. 2551.

[84]Ibid.

spending is on a collision course with economic realities.' "[85] While Canadian medical care uses up less GNP than the U.S. system, the expense of health care in Canada is one of the major factors in a Canadian federal per capita debt and per capita annual deficit that are twice as bad as those of the United States.[86]

The VA, Military Medicine, and Medicare/Medicaid: A Microcosm of Nationalized Health Care

Like many other health care experts, Stuart Wesbury believes that Americans would not accept the waiting lists, rationing, and other harassments found in national health care systems.[87] The problems are not unique to one country; they plague every national health system based on government funding. However, a student of such systems does not have to leave the United States to scrutinize the programs for such shortcomings, because they can be observed right here in our health programs: Medicare/Medicaid, military health care, and the Veterans' Administration.

Early in the Medicare program, Congress avoided the increasing-demand problem that resulted from implementation of the plan by simply spending whatever was necessary to pay for services (after imposing premiums and copayments). But as costs have ballooned out of control, Congress has been forced to apply increasing controls, such as limits on payments to hospitals and doctors and restrictions on coverage (rationing).

In the Department of Veterans' Affairs, with its own separate system of hospitals and physicians, the problems are more like those of Britain—chronic misallocation of resources and poor-quality patient care. Recent media exposés of poor-quality care in VA facilities, such as the hidden-camera observations within a VA hospital by the television show "Primetime Live" in September 1990, have shocked the nation.

"Primetime Live" found blood-stained needles lying on tables and equipment that was old and in disrepair in the VA hospital in Cleveland, Ohio. Veterans told the television crew that the nurses

---

[85]William E. Goodman, "The Canadian Model: Could It Work Here?" paper presented at the 46th annual meeting of the Association of American Physicians and Surgeons, Orlando, Florida, September 21, 1989.

[86]Ibid.

[87]Wesbury, "Why Other Nations' Rx Won't Work."

hadn't shaved or bathed them—one said for three weeks. Several had been lying in their own feces for hours. One hospital employee was quoted as noting, "Bad facilities, incompetent doctors, and medications that are ordered but don't get there."[88] Some of the nurses told the crew that doctors didn't change their gloves and routinely spread dangerous bacterial—staph—infections.[89]

The television show placed a hidden camera in the room of patient Charles Smith, a Vietnam veteran who had come into the hospital complaining of severe pain. According to nurses and staff, he did not receive prompt treatment, and as a result, surgery became necessary. His family accused the hospital of failing to treat his spinal abscess in time, and now Mr. Smith is paralyzed. The television camera showed that, although food was brought to Smith, no effort was made to feed him (he is a quadriplegic), and he went without food for three days—until a fellow patient wandered into his room and fed him.[90]

Patients at the Washington, D.C., VA Medical Center sometimes "walk around with a catheter for three or four months" awaiting prostate surgery, stated Chief of Medicine James Finkelstein. "It makes them vulnerable to infection and discomfort," he said and added that "we're doing the same thing they do in Great Britain."[91] John Peterson, 68, a World War II veteran, had all his upper teeth pulled by the Denver VA in September 1988, but he didn't receive his dentures until the following July. By then, his gums had shrunk, and the dentures had to be refitted. He finally received his dentures in November 1989.[92]

The New York Times recently reported that six men treated at the VA Medical Center in North Chicago during 1989 and 1990 died because of inadequate care.[93] Two died from undiagnosed ruptured aneurysms, one from undiagnosed heart blockage, one from hemorrhage following surgery, one from a misdiagnosed ulcer, and one

[88]ABC, "Primetime Live," transcript, September 27, 1990, p. 4.

[89]Ibid., p. 8.

[90]Ibid., pp. 5–6.

[91]Quoted in Janet Novack, "Hands off My Pork Barrel," Forbes, May 28, 1990, p. 183.

[92]Ibid.

[93]"U.S. Tells How 6 Died from Poor Care in Hospital," New York Times, April 10, 1991.

from an artery nicked during prostate surgery. During one of the emergency surgeries to repair a ruptured aneurysm, a small intestine was torn by a clamp and an artery was torn. The torn artery was not discovered until the autopsy. The man who died from heart blockage was given Maalox for suspected indigestion. A doctor noted the hemorrhaging of the man who had vocal cord surgery, but nothing was done to stop the bleeding, and he died.

Instead of realizing that the system itself is the root of the problem, however, media investigators such as those on "Primetime Live" concluded that deficiencies were caused by lack of funding. The plight of VA patients is eased only by the availability of alternative private insurance and hospitals for veterans unwilling to accept the inadequacies of the system.

The military health care system, which is similar to the VA system in that it uses its own separate system of hospitals and physicians, faces some of the same accusations as the VA—poor patient care and allocation of resources. One member of an active-duty family I spoke with remarked that the system is "okay if you never get very sick." A retired military officer told me that he avoided using the system when he was on active duty.[94]

Physicians who have practiced in the military have numerous concerns about the system, including lower standards of care, inequity of treatment of officers and enlisted personnel, rationing, quality assurance, constant movement of patients and doctors, bureaucratic red tape, and hassles with commanding officers who are not physicians. One physician I spoke with stated that the military system was "a prime example of socialized medicine," and another remarked that "with free care, you get what you pay for." Interestingly, many of the concerns listed by physicians are the same deficiencies found in nationalized health care systems—lower standards of care, inequity, rationing, lower quality, and bureaucracy.

State-Mandated Insurance Coverage

Although some politicians and organizations continue to push for national health care, a few states (Hawaii, Massachusetts, Oregon, and Washington) have already passed mini-versions of such

[94]From correspondence with the author.

a program, mandating universal health care coverage for all residents.

Hawaii

Adopted by the state of Hawaii in 1974, the program requires that employers cover all employees who work 20 or more hours per week for at least 4 consecutive weeks. Employers must pay at least 50 percent of premium costs, and employee premiums are limited to 1.5 percent of annual wages. The state subsidizes premiums paid by firms with fewer than eight employees.

Oregon

In 1989 the Oregon legislature passed the Oregon Basic Health Services Act, a program that is supposed to provide universal access to a basic level of care. It expands Medicaid eligibility, provides coverage for the medically uninsurable through a high-risk pool, and requires that employers provide insurance for all permanent employees and their dependents. Costs are shared by employers and employees, and there is a minimum required benefit level.

In an experiment with rationing, the program created a Health Services Commission that is in the process of prioritizing health services using criteria based on social values and the degree to which each service or procedure will benefit the health of the "entire" population. In March 1991 the program released a prioritized list of 700-plus health services. Following its release, the Oregon legislature decided to draw the line at medical service no. 587 in order to pay for health coverage of 120,000 uninsured residents. Some of the services deemed "nonessential" include treatment for acne, myasthenia gravis, tendinitis, chronic bronchitis, acute tonsillitis, and metastatic cancer with less than a 10 percent five-year survival rate. The state hopes to put the plan into effect in 1992 but will need a waiver from federal Medicaid rules.[95]

Washington

Washington State's Basic Health Plan is a demonstration project that was started in 1990 and is designed to provide health care coverage to up to 25,000 uninsured Washington residents. Those

[95]The above account is based on two sources: "Taking from the Poor and the Sick," *AAPS News* 47, no. 7 (July 1991); and "Oregon Cuts Funding for 122 Medical Services," *AAPS News* 47 no. 8 (August 1991).

who are eligible pay reduced monthly premiums, based on family size and income, for health care coverage through private-sector providers.[96] The plan contracts with privately managed health care systems to provide a basic benefit package for a set monthly rate. The plan pays the costs of the program with a mixture of premiums and state revenues. No deductible is charged.

Massachusetts

At the request of then-governor Michael Dukakis, the state of Massachusetts passed legislation in 1988 that was intended to provide all residents with health insurance beginning in 1992. Under the Massachusetts law, the cost of mandatory health insurance is shared by businesses and employees, with businesses paying into a state insurance pool. If a company already has insurance benefits for its workers, it can deduct the premiums from the surcharge. By 1992 companies were to pay a maximum annual surcharge of $1,680 per worker to fund the state pool. Companies with fewer than six employees were to be exempt.[97]

Does Lack of Health Insurance Equal Lack of Health Care?

The primary focus of the existing state plans is on providing access to health care insurance—a view that assumes that those without insurance lack access to health care. However, an analysis of the Massachusetts Health Plan by Dr. Attiat F. Ott and Dr. Wayne Gray indicates that this assumption is flawed.[98]

On a nationwide basis, according to Ott and Gray, approximately 18 percent of the population is not covered by either public or private insurance. This incidence of uninsurance is found in every selected population group, not just in the unemployed and working

---

[96]The plan is available in selected demonstration areas to people who are under the age of 65, who do not qualify for Medicare, and who have a gross family income that does not exceed 200 percent of the federal poverty level (the poverty level is currently $25,400 for a family of four).

[97]Recently, the newly elected governor of Massachusetts signed into law a three-year delay on the implementation of the employer-mandate portion of the plan. Gov. William Weld actually wants repeal of the entire plan, but small businesses asked for the delay because they believed that repeal (although they support it) would not have been possible before the January 1992 deadline for implementation of the employer mandate.

[98]Attiat F. Ott and Wayne B. Gray, *The Massachusetts Health Plan: The Right Prescription?* (Boston: Pioneer Institute for Public Policy Research, 1988), chap. 2.

poor. Furthermore, the numbers are almost identical for men and women (18.1 percent and 18.2 percent, respectively); singles have a higher rate of uninsurance than married (24.1 percent versus 11.4 percent); and nonwhite citizens have a higher rate of uninsurance than white citizens (34.3 percent and 15.7 percent).[99]

Forty-two percent of the uninsured nationwide fall into the 25–64 age group. Seventy-one percent of those uninsured are not married. Forty-eight percent of the uninsured are employed, and 51.8 percent have an annual family income of $5,000–$20,000. Fifteen percent of those uninsured have yearly family incomes of over $50,000.[100]

In Massachusetts almost 60 percent of the uninsured were from families that earned more than $20,000 a year.[101] Presumably this uninsured population could have paid for health insurance but for some reason has chosen not to. However, according to Ott and Gray's research, an individual is far more likely to be without insurance if he or she is unemployed, is in a family earning less than $20,000, and is nonwhite.[102]

The authors' most significant conclusion was that there was no convincing evidence that the uninsured lack access to adequate health care. In a National Health Interview Survey study conducted over a 12-month period, 27 percent of the insured population nationwide reported above-average physician visits (five visits), the same percentage reported by the uninsured.[103] Eighteen percent of those insured reported above-average hospital stays (average 12 days), while 22 percent of the uninsured had above-average stays.[104]

The conclusions reached by Ott and Gray indicate that the utilization of health services shows only slight differences between the insured and the uninsured populations. The authors determined that being uninsured was not necessarily detrimental to health care access in the United States.[105]

[99]Data cited by Ott and Gray are from the 1984 National Health Interview Survey.
[100]Ott and Gray, Table 2.9, p. 29.
[101]Ibid., Table 2.2, p. 17.
[102]Ibid., Table 2.9, p. 29.
[103]Ibid., Table 2.12, p. 33.
[104]Ibid.
[105]Ibid, p. 35.

Does State-Mandated Insurance Coverage Work?

The various state plans were enacted to achieve the noble goal of affording the uninsured access to medical care.[106] Ironically, although the plans were instituted to help those thought to be in need, in reality they are having a whole host of unintended and damaging effects on just those people—the uninsured, unemployed, and low-wage employees, as well as on employers and the economy in general.

Mandating insurance coverage by employers lowers the take-home pay of workers by requiring employers to substitute fringe benefits for wage income. It limits the choices of those workers who would rather receive their compensation in wages. The higher costs to employers of this type of program (estimated at $650 million for the Massachusetts Health Plan in 1992) will result in a loss of primarily low-wage jobs (an estimated 9,000 in Massachusetts).[107] Small employers of low-wage workers would be most affected; some would be put out of business, thereby adding to the numbers of unemployed.

Reductions in jobs and wages would result in lower state and federal payroll and income taxes, upsetting cost estimates for such programs and contributing to state and federal deficits. An unexpected recession or downturn in the economy could have devastating effects on unemployment and increase budgetary pressures on government programs. In Massachusetts a downturn in the state's economy has almost doubled the unemployment rate since 1988 and has already put the health care program in financial jeopardy.[108]

Under the Massachusetts plan, companies that do not currently offer health insurance are eligible for a tax credit to entice them into the program. That enticement has angered many small businesses that currently offer health insurance and now see their competitors

---

[106]According to Charles D. Baker, assistant secretary of health for the state of Massachusetts, even though the Massachusetts Health Plan was enacted to provide health insurance for the uninsured, only 10–15 percent of the approximately 100,000 unemployed are covered under the plan.

[107]Charles D. Baker, "The Massachusetts Debacle," paper presented by the Pioneer Institute before the National Federation of Independent Business Foundation, Washington, April 5, 1990, p. 8.

[108]From correspondence with Charles D. Baker, Massachusetts assistant secretary of health.

being rewarded for their delay in offering benefits. Any Massachusetts small business that currently offers health insurance is paying income, property, and sales taxes to finance discounted health insurance coverage to competitors who have not provided coverage in the past.

The payroll tax required in Massachusetts (12 percent on each worker's first $14,000 in wages, which can be waived by purchasing at least $1,680 worth of health care coverage) hits low- and middle-income workers the hardest. They are the most likely to lose their jobs, and because payroll taxes ultimately come out of wages (in the form of lower wages), $1,680 hurts a low-income worker more than the worker making $50,000 annually.

Setting a particular dollar amount on benefits or mandating a specific type of coverage eliminates workers' freedom of choice by forcing them to accept health insurance even if they don't want it or by mandating a higher level of coverage than the individual worker would like. A worker who wants to purchase a no-frills insurance plan is not given that choice because the employer is not allowed to offer it or is penalized for doing so.

Furthermore, the Massachusetts program sets up the incentive for companies to drop the insurance they're currently offering in favor of a government-provided program. The same design flaw exists in the Washington Basic Health Plan. With the state offering low-cost health care coverage for workers, what incentive do employers have to keep offering health insurance?

Because of tight qualifications in the unemployment insurance portion of the Massachusetts program, some workers may not qualify for the plan and will remain uninsured. For example, a man who works in Massachusetts but lives in New Hampshire would pay into the program. If he were laid off his job, he would not qualify for benefits because he is not a Massachusetts resident. On the other hand, a man who lives in Massachusetts and works in New Hampshire would not pay into the program, but he would receive benefits in Massachusetts.

And finally, higher labor costs due to the additional costs of providing coverage for workers and paying the increased payroll taxes will make it more difficult for U.S. companies to compete in world markets. A comparison with Europe, where mandated benefits and other controls on business are a permanent feature, shows the economic results on competitiveness. Since 1970 the United States has created 34 million new jobs; over the same period, Europe—with a population 50 percent larger than that of the United States—has added only 2 million jobs.[109]

Congressional Proposals for Mandated Insurance Coverage

As of May 1992 there were 800 pieces of legislation dealing with health care issues before Congress. Some promote the adoption of a national health care system, such as the comprehensive cradle-to-grave plan proposed by Rep. Pete Stark (D-Calif.), that would cost $120 billion a year and be financed in part by a 4 percent tax on all income over $16,000. Others tinker with the current hodgepodge of programs, and some, such as the 1989 bill put forward by Sen. Edward Kennedy (D-Mass.), introduce mandated employer insurance ("play-or-pay") on the national level. According to the 1990 Metropolitan Life survey (conducted by Louis Harris and Associates), 50 percent of health-care leaders questioned believed that by the year 2000 the United States will have a federal law requiring all employers to provide health insurance for their employees.[110]

The Minimum Health Benefits for All Workers Act

The Minimum Health Benefits for All Workers Act (S.768 and H.R. 1845) was introduced by Sen. Edward Kennedy and Rep. Henry Waxman (D-Calif.) in early 1989. Under the plan, each employer would have to enroll in a minimum health insurance plan all employees working more than 17 hours a week. Employees would not be allowed to waive participation in the health plan unless covered by their working spouse. A minimum benefit package would be established, and the insurance plan could not exclude coverage for anyone with a preexisting condition. The plan would have a small deductible and would cover at least 80 percent of costs after the deductible was met. The plan also has to provide

[109]John C. Goodman, Gary Robbins, and Aldona Robbins, *Mandating Health Insurance*, NCPA Policy Report no. 136 (Dallas: National Center for Policy Analysis, February 1989), p. 18.

[110]"Trade-offs & Choices: Health Policy Options for the 1990s," a survey conducted for Metropolitan Life Insurance Company by Louis Harris and Associates, New York, 1990.

catastrophic coverage, paying all costs once the worker has spent $3,000 out of pocket.

Under the Kennedy bill, employers would have to pay at least 80 percent of the premiums, and cover 100 percent for low-wage workers. Employers with fewer than 25 employees and without a health plan would have to purchase insurance through a "regional insurer." The secretary of health and human services would establish several health insurance "regions." The secretary would then certify a number of insurers to offer a minimum benefit package in those regions.

Effects of the Kennedy Bill

According to an analysis done by economists John C. Goodman, Gary Robbins, and Aldona Robbins, the Kennedy bill would impose on the private sector a cost of at least $108 billion and possibly as high as $159 billion in its first year of operation.[111] Approximately two-thirds of the cost of the program would stem from the need to expand coverage for workers already insured to meet the mandated benefit requirements, even though the focus of the proposed legislation is to provide coverage for those who are uninsured. As discussed previously, higher employer costs come out of employee wages, resulting in lower take-home pay, increased unemployment, and reduced productivity. Estimates are that there would be as many as 1.1 million fewer jobs and as much as $27 billion in lower productivity nationwide attributable to implementation of the Kennedy bill.

Goodman, Robbins, and Robbins have calculated that the Kennedy bill would raise health care costs by at least $108 billion in its first year of operation. Based on a $250 deductible, and the annual premiums of $1,465 for individuals and $3,529 for families called for in the bill, the cost of new coverage (for those currently uninsured) would be $37.3 billion; the increased cost of existing coverage (the minimum insurance package specified in the bill is more expensive than what most employers currently provide) would be $68 billion; and additional administrative costs (costs incurred by small employers forced to offer insurance) would be $3 billion. The higher demand that would ensue from government-required mandates

---

[111]The findings in this section are drawn primarily from the Goodman, Robbins, and Robbins study, pp. 9–16.

would result in even higher health care prices for everyone. The plan would also increase the federal deficit through decreased tax revenues (estimated at $46.5 billion) resulting from the fallout loss of jobs and increased unemployment compensation.

Like the state-mandated insurance plans mentioned above, the Kennedy bill would eliminate the worker's freedom of choice. Employees would be forced to accept a plan they might not want, and employees of small businesses would be further restricted because their employer would have to choose coverage from a regional insurer.

The Kennedy bill also would place a disproportionate burden on small businesses, which may currently offer minimal or no health benefits. As they are already struggling to compete with larger companies, the cost of providing mandated health coverage could force some of them out of business, thereby contributing to unemployment.

Finally, legislating a minimum package of benefits extends an invitation to every special-interest lobbyist to pressure Washington for additions to the benefits package. With the inevitable growth of benefits, program costs would soar, contributing to the vicious cycle of higher employer costs and unemployment.

The Pepper Commission and Its Call for Action

The Pepper Commission, or the U.S. Bipartisan Commission on Comprehensive Health Care, was named for the late Rep. Claude Pepper (D-Fla.). Its mission was to recommend legislation that would ensure that all Americans would have coverage for health care and long-term care. The commission, consisting of six senators, six representatives, and three presidential appointees, released its report, *A Call for Action*, in September 1990.

The commission recommended adoption of a combination of a federally mandated health insurance and a nationalized health care system that would include the following:

- A phased-in system of mandatory employer coverage for all workers. Tax credits would be provided for small business; low-income workers and the unemployed would receive subsidies toward their contribution; and a federal program would be instituted to provide insurance for companies that wanted it.

117

- Mandatory coverage for all individuals from their employer or from the public program.
- Expansion and replacement of the Medicaid system with a federal program.
- A federally specified minimum benefit package, with deductibles or copayments, that would cover preventive and primary care and hospital care.
- Formulation of national practice guidelines and standards of care that would increase regulation and control of physicians. Development of a uniform price schedule, with local organizations formed and held accountable for quality assurance and assessment.
- Development of a comprehensive public insurance program for all long-term care services.

The estimated first-year cost for this program (based on 1990 figures) is $70 billion, including $12 billion for the mandatory employer coverage and federalization of Medicaid and $42 billion for the long-term care program. Although the commission offered no specifics on how to fund the proposal, it announced that to finance the first year through new taxes would require $430 from every nonpoor adult. The commission did recommend that taxes be progressive and grow fast enough to keep up with benefit growth (and increased demand) and that contributions come from people of all ages.

The insurance sections of the proposal that require mandatory employer coverage would have the same harmful effects on employees, employers, and the economy as the proposed Kennedy legislation. According to Rep. Bill Gradison (R-Ohio), a dissenter on the report, "Costs of $3,000 to $4,000 a year for each worker are neither uncommon nor trivial in amount. In my view, the Commission consistently understates the costs of health insurance today. In some cases, this increase in employers' payments for workers will cost jobs."[112]

The increased regulation and control of physicians and their practices and fees would amount to the socialization of doctors,

[112]Excerpts from a letter from Representative Gradison to Sen. Jay Rockefeller (D-W.Va.), chairman of the Pepper Commission. The letter appeared on the editorial page of the *Wall Street Journal*, March 8, 1990.

with the concomitant effects already found in Canada—physician dissatisfaction, demoralization, increased rates of early retirement, and other losses from the profession.

The economic effect of transferring millions of people to a federal program would be an ever-increasing demand for additional benefits, opening the floodgates for lobbyists and special-interest groups alike to hound Congress for more goodies. As Gradison understands: "Over 100 million Americans would then look to the federal government for their health insurance. As a result, the political pressures to increase benefits would likely result in costs to taxpayers far above what even the Commission estimates."[113]

AmeriCare

AmeriCare is the legislative proposal that developed out of the Pepper Commission report. Introduced in June 1991 by Senate majority leader George Mitchell (D-Me.) and coauthored by Sens. Edward Kennedy (D-Mass.), Donald Reigle (D-Mich.), and Jay Rockefeller (D-W.Va.), the bill incorporates all of the important steps emphasized by the Pepper Commission.

Under the plan, all employers would be required either to provide coverage meeting basic standards for their workers and their families or to contribute a percentage of their payroll to a new public insurance program called AmeriCare. AmeriCare would replace the current Medicaid system and would insure anyone not covered by an employer plan. People under the poverty line wouldn't have to pay a premium, and those above would pay at a rate based on their income.

Under the plan, there would be a basic package of covered services that would be the same for those covered by employers or by the AmeriCare program. Mitchell has estimated the cost to the federal government at $6 billion for the first year, with a cost savings of almost $80 billion in health expenditures over the following five years.[114]

To curb health costs, the bill calls for an independent board that would set national spending goals for health care by negotiating with representatives of various sectors of health care. Unnecessary

[113]Ibid.

[114]"HealthAmerica: Affordable Health Care for All Americans," a document released by the office of Senate majority leader George Mitchell, June 5, 1991.

care would be reduced (that is, rationed) by (1) a program of outcomes research to determine what care is necessary or unnecessary, (2) development of practice guidelines to assist physicians in providing only necessary care and to assist insurers in deciding what care should be reimbursed, and (3) an enhanced program of technology assessment to help determine the usefulness of expensive medical techniques. The bill also recommends granting tax breaks to small businesses and individuals to help them buy health insurance. The plan would be phased in over five years, with smaller businesses being given time to comply with the mandatory insurance regulations.

Many of the same detrimental effects of the Kennedy legislation, the Pepper Commission recommendations, and the Dukakis plan in Massachusetts are to be found in the AmeriCare plan. As in the Massachusetts plan, increased unemployment would result because small businesses could not afford the health insurance mandates, even with tax credits. Reductions in federal and state tax revenues due to higher unemployment would increase the cost estimates for the AmeriCare program.

Mandating a specific package of benefits reduces freedom of choice for individuals in their purchase of health insurance. Instituting a government program with a mandated package of benefits would stimulate a feeding frenzy of special-interest lobbyists who will flock to Washington, their only purpose being to expand the number of mandated benefits to include their sponsors' services.

Depending on how the payroll tax was structured, in some cases it could be more beneficial for companies already offering health coverage to drop it and thereby dump their employees onto the public plan. The phase-in portions of the legislation would still leave workers uninsured if they were employed by small businesses, and those workers would be added to the AmeriCare rolls. Most likely, they would stay there even after the deadline for employer-provided insurance passed. The Office of Management and Budget estimates that 45 percent of the population—an increase from approximately 25 percent in 1991—would gradually be transferred to the public health plan by 1996 if a play-or-pay program were enacted.[115]

[115]From a speech by Tom Scully, assistant director, Office of Management and Budget, at a National Chamber Foundation conference on health care, Washington, November 14, 1991.

Deciding what care is necessary or unnecessary and limiting the use of technology—both currently part of the Canadian system—are forms of rationing. Such limitations, combined with the increased regulation of physicians, will result in the same physician dissatisfaction, early retirement, and career changes by doctors that have occurred in Canada.

The idea of establishing national spending targets is taken directly from the Canadian system. The targets would be designed with "voluntary" spending limits for the total amount spent on doctors' fees and hospital services across the country. However, because one cannot expect thousands of physicians and hospitals acting independently to agree on specific targets, such voluntary limits would soon become mandatory.

The American College of Physicians' Plan

The proposal by the American College of Physicians (ACP) would have two elements: (1) a play-or-pay, employer-mandated insurance system for all employees and their dependents and (2) a government-based insurance program that would replace Medicare, Medicaid, and other federal programs and would cover all uninsured workers. ACP would mandate a universal-coverage benefit plan that includes "medically effective and other health-related services that society values."[116]

Financing for the plan would be as follows: (1) employers would pay 50 percent of premiums (play) or 6 percent of payroll (pay), plus a 3 percent corporate income tax; (2) employees would pay up to 50 percent of premiums or 6 percent of wages, plus a 3 percent personal income tax; (3) the poor and self-employed who earn up to 200 percent of the poverty level amount would make contributions on a sliding scale, beginning at zero and rising to a maximum of one-half the public program cost; and (4) people over age 60 would pay, after a transition, premiums that would eventually be means tested and limited to one-half the public program cost at 200 percent of poverty.

The ACP proposal recommends instituting national physician practice guidelines, which would determine what treatment was

---

[116]"Universal Health Care: A Plan for Change," draft proposal by the American College of Physicians, July 1991, p. 6.

"medically appropriate," and it recommends setting "appropriate prices" for medical services by adopting the resource-based relative-value scale for *all* physicians.[117] The plan would control the supply and distribution of health care professionals by offering training funds or forgiving loans to "enhance variably the supply of specialties and the geographic distribution of physicians."[118]

The ACP claims that although its plan would provide universal coverage with a minimum package of benefits, the total cost of such a program would be less than that of our current system. However, ACP contradicts itself by stating, "We believe that under the proposal, total costs to most employers and to individuals will not increase and that in many cases they will decrease, but government's revenues (through employer pay-ins and increases in corporate and personal income tax rates) will increase."[119] How can the costs to business and individuals decrease when government revenues are increasing?

The ACP responds that there will be savings on premium and out-of-pocket costs that will lower costs to businesses and individuals. But for many employees, premium costs will increase because many employers currently cover most of the premium cost, whereas under this plan employee contributions could rise to 50 percent. And as mentioned with regard to other play-or-pay plans, the demand to expand the minimum benefit package would eventually negate any savings. Many workers, who already have good coverage through their employers, do not suffer significant out-of-pocket costs. While a few might benefit from lower out-of-pocket costs, under such a plan most taxpayers would see an overall increase in their taxes.

The Drift toward National Health Care

Many of the people dealing with health care issues, both inside and outside government, believe that the never-ending budget and federal deficit crisis plaguing Washington, D.C., will thwart any attempts to adopt some kind of national health care system. They say that we should not worry, that the costs are too great, and that

---

[117]The resource-based relative-value scale will be discussed in detail later.

[118]"Universal Health Care," p. 10.

[119]Ibid., p. 12.

Congress and the White House will never agree on how to raise the massive amounts of revenue necessary to fund such a system.

And there are others in the nation's capital who agree; they say that the American public probably will never turn on C-SPAN and watch an up-or-down vote by members of Congress on nationalized health care. However, those experts disagree that our system of health care will never be nationalized. In fact, they'll tell you that it's happening right now and that, if the trends continue, America will probably have nationalized health care by the end of the century.

How is that possible? Well, it all started gradually during the 1960s when we instituted a system of national health care for our elderly and poor (Medicare and Medicaid) and expanded services for veterans (Veterans' Administration programs) and Native Americans (Indian Health Service programs). A blizzard of regulations during the 1970s and 1980s has dulled our senses and desensitized us to federal control. Use of the prospective payment system, which sets a fixed schedule of fees paid to hospitals for treatment of Medicare patients for 475 diagnostic related groups, means that hospitals already deliver care within a predetermined budget.

Health maintenance organizations, which were developed during the 1970s and 1980s, introduced doctors to additional regulation of the practice of medicine and conditioned patients to expect someone else to pay for their care (third-party payment). The professional standards review organizations conditioned physicians to the idea of someone else's reviewing their work and deciding what treatment is appropriate and whether it meets certain standards.

With the 1990s came a new rung in the government ladder of control of health care: the resource-based relative-value scale (RBRVS). The RBRVS replaced the system of "usual, customary, and reasonable" charges that had been adopted by Medicare in 1965 and by many other payers after that. The RBRVS is based on the relative value of resources that would typically be expended to provide a given service—in other words, the time and effort doctors actually devote to each procedure. The new fee schedule took effect on January 1, 1992.

The RBRVS includes geographical adjustment factors to reflect differences in practice costs, malpractice costs, and work components. The primary factors used to determine the relative value scale are the amount of time and the intensity of effort needed to produce each service. The new payment schedule means higher fees for doctors in such specialties as family practice, internal medicine, and obstetrics, and lower fees for surgeons and radiologists.

Researchers at Harvard University worked with several medical groups, including the AMA, to reach agreement on a system that physicians believed fairly measured the relative resource value of different medical services within their own specialties. The researchers categorized the resources that differentiated the services into relative values. They gathered extensive data on the amount of time and the intensity of effort needed to perform many medical procedures. The data were combined with information from other sources and analyzed using a formula to develop the relative-value scale of services within 18 medical specialties.

A second part of the RBRVS plan imposes a complicated formula for calculating how much fees will rise each year. In addition, the legislation will limit balance billing, the amount doctors can charge above what Medicare allows for a procedure or office visit.

An Analysis of RBRVS

During the 1980s the concept of comparable worth gained increasing attention from many in Washington, D.C., and across the country. Several pieces of legislation were introduced at the national level, and a few states were also interested in the idea. Comparable-worth proponents make the argument that the market does not fairly reimburse people for their work efforts and that someone else (that is, the government) must intervene to remedy this so-called mistake. The RBRVS, in reality, is nothing more than a comparable-worth program for physicians.

Under comparable worth, the wage levels for federal jobs held predominantly by women would be compared to those for jobs held predominantly by men. Any gap in pay found after factoring out "objective" job criteria—such as complexity, knowledge needed, judgment, and amount of discretion required—would be attributed to sex discrimination and corrected. This valuation could serve as a model for private-sector job evaluations. Under the RBRVS, the system is essentially the same, except that comparisons are made among physician specialties.

The concept of comparable worth, or the RBRVS, is alien to the free-market system, in which supply and demand have always been the best instruments for determining prices, including the price of labor. Labor is not exempt from the same market forces that determine the prices of other commodities. The recent collapse of the command economy of the Soviet Union, where all prices were set by government decree, is a shining example of why price setting does not work. The Soviet government, which set prices after studying market prices in the West, always lagged behind because bureaucracy-set prices can never react quickly enough to the prices set by hundreds of millions of consumers as they make decisions in the marketplace.

As were the price-setting procedures in the Soviet command system, even a yearly revaluation of the RBRVS would be far too slow to account for changes in the personal preferences of medical consumers. In addition to the fact that one person may value a surgeon's skill over his or her family physician's bedside manner while another may not, many other factors go into the prices charged by physicians (such as years of schooling, specialization, residencies and internships, and cost of medical school). Those who attend 12 years of medical school to become ophthalmologists, delaying their earning power by several years, have traditionally commanded higher fees in the marketplace than general practitioners, who spend far less time and money in training.

Comparable worth, or pay equity, as it is now called, has not fared well in Congress. Although numerous attempts have been made, no legislation incorporating the concept has passed both the Senate and the House. In Canada, the province of Ontario, faced with a new law on pay equity, has been wrestling with how to compare the jobs done by people as diverse as secretaries and warehouse workers, janitors and telephone operators.[120] While the Ontario Pay Equity Commission provides guidelines for determining pay equity, companies and government departments must draw up their own plans for rectifying any inequities. Many employers, including the provincial government itself, have had difficulty deciding on valuations for their jobs and are missing the law's deadlines. Some employees are angry with the valuations. For example, Toronto nurses were annoyed at being equated with

---

[120]Lynne Kilpatrick, "In Ontario, 'Equal Pay for Equal Work' Becomes a Reality, but Not Very Easily," *Wall Street Journal*, March 9, 1990.

chefs, and both secretaries and truck drivers were offended at being found equal. At the University of Toronto, pay-equity changes left some accountants earning less than the clerks they supervise.[121]

Given the political failure of the comparable-worth idea for U.S. government workers, the difficulty that Ontario is having implementing its pay-equity scheme, and the obvious failure of a national system of setting prices in the Soviet Union, why would the U.S. government want to adopt such a program for paying its Medicare physicians? Such a system would surely skew the demand for various types of physicians; the government might encourage more students to become family practitioners and fewer to become surgeons. But isn't it the job of the market to decide the supply of physicians based on demand? If the central planners in Moscow could not get bread to the grocery stores, how can we expect that well-meaning U.S. planners would correctly decide how many radiologists and gynecologists we should have?

Many health care experts in the nation's capital believe that the proponents of nationalized health care view the RBRVS simply as the next step toward a totally nationalized system. Those experts fear that after the RBRVS is in place, private insurance companies will adopt it for their reimbursement schedules. In fact, according to Kenneth Bacon of the *Wall Street Journal*, the RBRVS "is expected to be adopted as the basis for payment by private insurance companies."[122]

Some health care analysts believe that implementation of the RBRVS will result in many physicians' dropping their Medicare patients. Already, a visit by a Medicare patient generates as many as 10 pieces of paper for the physician to fill out. Accordingly, if the prices that physicians can charge are further limited, they may find it necessary to drop such patients because they can't afford to treat them. If that happens, the next step in the process will be the mandatory assigning of Medicare doctors (a bill proposing this has already been introduced by Rep. Brian Donnelly [D-Mass.]).

[121]Ibid.

[122]Kenneth H. Bacon, "Plan to Overhaul Payment of Doctors Under Medicare Is Agreed to by Conferees," *Wall Street Journal*, November 21, 1989. In early 1992, Rep. Dan Rostenkowski (D-Ill.) introduced legislation to apply the RBRVS reimbursement schedules to physicians treating non-Medicare patients.

Physicians would be forced to accept Medicare patients whether they wanted to or not.

In a 1990 survey by the Association of American Physicians and Surgeons, doctors responded that several proposed and actual changes in the Medicare system would affect their ability to continue accepting Medicare patients: 47 percent would restrict the number of their Medicare patients because of a ban on balance billing, 47 percent would restrict their Medicare patient load because of cuts in reimbursement, 56 percent would restrict their load because of mandatory assignment, and 57 percent would reduce that load following adoption of federal practice guidelines.[123]

If we are to complete the U.S. voyage to national health care, all that is needed is passage of a mandatory employer insurance program (the Kennedy or AmeriCare proposal), mandatory control of drugs and drug prices (as proposed in a bill introduced in 1991 by Sen. David Pryor [D-Ark.]), and federal certification of physicians (as proposed in 1991 by Rep. Pete Stark [D-Calif.]). The public health system is already testing a new program of federal practice guidelines for physicians, and those could be used to mandate how all physicians could practice.

So, like a thief in the night, a nationalized health care system could creep up on the American people, without that up-or-down vote on C-SPAN or a national referendum.

Freedom of Choice Is the Alternative

Obviously, the concept of a national system of health care is not new to the world, in that most countries do have such a system. However, as has been detailed in this chapter, the inadequacies of such programs are that they provide less than high-quality care for their citizens at costs that are out of control because of the lack of attention given the laws of economics.

The basic defect that afflicts such programs across the board, the Canadian system as well as the Kennedy proposal, is that they all fail to account for the ability of the marketplace to provide freedom of choice for both the consumer and the provider of services. Americans believe in the "market" for most of the other transactions they undertake in their daily lives. Why not for health care? People in other countries, particularly those in Eastern Europe, will be quick

[123]*AAPS News* 46, no. 5 (May 1990).

to state that government control over people's lives and decision-making doesn't work. If it doesn't work when control is exerted over every aspect of life, why should we expect it to work in selected areas? And why would it be prudent for the United States to adopt a national system of health care just because most other countries have one?

Because the majority of American citizens are insured and generally satisfied with their health care, there is no compelling reason for throwing the baby out with the bath water and adopting a national health care program to ensure that the small number of uninsured receives coverage. The correct answer to spiraling costs and lack of health insurance is to use the market, the only mechanism that provides freedom of consumer choice. The question remaining is, How do we get there from here?

The crazy quilt of health care programs created by both the federal and state governments has virtually destroyed the American people's access to reasonable and efficient health care. Only the elimination of government interference—that is, creating a free market in health care—will end the move toward nationalization. Only a free market will break the spiral of ever-increasing medical costs. As economist Ludwig von Mises wrote, "The pricing process of the unhampered market directs production into those channels in which it best serves the wishes of the consumers as manifested on the market."[124] Only a free market in health care will allow individuals a maximum amount of choice in meeting their health care needs.

So, how *do* we get there from here?

[124]Ludwig von Mises, *Human Action: A Treatise on Economics* (Chicago: Contemporary Books, 1966), p. 394.

5. Health Care Based on Consumer Choice

How do we stop the downward spiral toward nationalized health care, with all its concomitant defects, and instead embrace a system that trusts the decisions of individuals? How do we extract ourselves from the ever-deepening hole in which we find our health care system and transform that system to one grounded on consumer choice and the market?

Changes to Improve the Health Care System

Initially, both politicians and the general public must undergo a behavioral and attitudinal transformation to make positive change a reality. Following that, reforms must be enacted to smooth the transition to a system based on market operations and freedom of choice.

First, and probably most difficult, Congress must adopt a long-term outlook on health care. To satisfy voters and win reelection, most politicians opt for the short-term fix to problems. Members of Congress need to step back and consider a comprehensive approach to reforming the health care system, putting a halt to the piecemeal regulation and control that have served only to complicate and confound an already deteriorating condition.

Second, Americans must not fear changes in their health care system. They are wary that reform will leave them worse off, and their apprehension fosters resistance to any modifications in the current structure. An electorate educated and informed on the benefits of reform will ensure the reform's political success. Advocates of change, therefore, should explain its value to the public.

Third, Congress and the public alike must realize that a market can function in the field of health care. Conventional wisdom espouses the idea that health care is not subject to normal economic laws of competition governing the supply of goods and services. There is a claim that health care is too fundamental a good to be

129

left to the market. But the same can be said for clothes and food, yet their production and distribution are predominately left to the market. Pundits announce that consumers are not capable of making informed decisions about their medical care without assistance from Big Brother. In reality, consumers lack a basic understanding of many of the services they contract for, but that lack does not prevent them from enlisting the aid of an auto mechanic, an appliance repairman, or an attorney on a regular basis.

Consumers compensate for their lack of knowledge by asking friends for recommendations or by consulting consumer magazines. Most consumers shop around, receiving price quotes and asking what kind of service will be provided. The process is similar with medical care. If people need a doctor, they generally ask friends or relatives for a recommendation, or they contact their family doctor if a specialist is needed. Furthermore, if a special procedure or operation is recommended, many patients will obtain a second opinion.

Critics say that a market may operate adequately for routine care, but when faced with an emergency, patients do not have time to comparison shop. In actuality, most medical emergencies are covered by insurance, and even here a market functions as consumers shop around for insurance that provides the coverage they need at the price they want. In any case, medical emergencies account for only 15 percent of all medical care.[1]

Proponents of national health care often remark that the United States has already tried a market system in health care and it has failed. However, as the historical look at the development of health care presented in Chapter 3 shows, the problems plaguing the current system are not the fault of a free market. In this century, America has never really seen a free market in health care. Rather, the market has been controlled through government regulation and interference, which have distorted any normal market signals by which consumers and providers could make decisions regarding affordable, efficient health care.

Fourth, the consumers of health care must be willing to assume personal responsibility for their own care. As the saying goes, "You

[1]Rita Ricardo-Campbell, *The Economics and Politics of Health Care* (Chapel Hill: University of North Carolina Press, 1982), p. 93.

can't get something for nothing." For too long, consumers have expected someone else—the third-party payer—to pay for their health care. But, as shown in Chapter 3, that system has been fundamentally responsible for the meteoric rise in health care costs. The best way to keep health care costs under control is to *increase* freedom of choice and personal responsibility. According to Otto H. Nowotny, director of F. Hoffman-La Roche, a pharmaceutical company:

> Personal responsibility in healthcare matters must therefore be encouraged wherever possible, and the nearly century-old tradition of having governments assume the burden for even the most trivial healthcare expenditure must be reversed. The proper economic signals must be given, such as direct and full payment by the patients themselves of a financially tolerable proportion of individual annual health-care expenses.[2]

Assuming individual responsibility must include bearing the costs and reaping the benefits of the lifestyles we choose. The most common measures of health that people want to see improved, such as life expectancy, are affected only marginally by health care. The effects of diet; way of life; personal habits; and even housing, education, crime, drugs, and poverty are far greater than the influence of health care. More and more health experts are realizing that health and life expectancy are influenced by lifestyle choices. Exercising freedom of choice in lifestyle also means accepting responsibility for the choices made. If one chooses to engage in behavior risky to one's health, such as smoking, one must be willing to accept the consequences. The failure to require people to bear the costs of their risky behavior only encourages it.

How do we solve the problem of rising health care costs? Solving the problem requires transferring the power of choice to individual consumers. It requires removing third parties from the payment system and establishing a direct relationship between the purchaser and the supplier of health care. It demands the removal of government controls and regulations that manipulate and distort the system. And it requires the assumption of individual responsibility,

---

[2]Otto Herbert Nowotny, "The Challenge Facing the Healthcare Industry in the 1990s," *Drugs Made in Germany* 33, 1 (1990): 3, 4.

whereby consumers are liable for their own behavior and spend their own money when they purchase medical care. The balance of this chapter offers detailed procedures for achieving those objectives.

Changes in Treatment of Individual Workers and Families

Tax incentives for employer-provided health insurance were encouraged during World War II, when wages were frozen and employers needed something to offer potential employees. Although that policy did result in greater access to health care for many Americans, it was a primary contributor to the ongoing inflation in health care prices. Having a third party pay for health care decreases an employee's incentive to control costs. The consumer is not interested in obtaining the best services for the dollar and does not realize that higher premiums result from this lack of concern about costs.

A first step toward encouraging consumers to become more prudent buyers of medical care is to make health insurance benefits part of the gross wage of employees and to allow tax credits for premiums on individual tax returns. Employees would then be allowed to choose a health insurance policy tailored to their individual and family needs. Allowing all individuals a tax credit for a portion of their health insurance premiums would correct a long-standing bias—those who have employer-provided health insurance can receive coverage while the self-employed and those working for small businesses often cannot afford coverage.

Such changes in the tax code would expand the availability of health insurance beyond those who work for large companies that offer benefits purchased with pretax dollars (money removed from their paycheck for health benefits and not included in taxable income). Currently, those who are self-employed or who work for small companies that cannot afford health benefits must pay for their health insurance with after-tax monies.

Offering the individual a tax credit would reduce the traditional opposition to eliminating the tax incentives for employer-provided insurance. Many fear that the loss of the employer tax incentives would increase workers' tax liability, but that concern would be removed by offering the incentives on the personal side of the tax code.

If they purchased the insurance themselves, consumers would become more cost conscious and would comparison shop for the best coverage at the most reasonable price. In addition, consumers could tailor their coverage to meet their individual needs. Often, workers find that they must choose from the few medical plans offered by their company, none of which fit their needs. People employed by small businesses often find their choices even more restricted than do those working for large corporations.

The tax credit could be limited to the amount of a no-frills, catastrophic-type policy. A relatively healthy person or family might want to purchase a catastrophic-only policy, at a lower premium, and pay for routine medical expenses out of pocket. The tax credit would cover this policy. A consumer or family that incurs more routine expenses might choose a more comprehensive policy, with a higher premium, and pay the amount above the deduction or credit.

Another advantage of individually purchased health insurance is that workers would be able to take their coverage with them as they changed jobs. Changes in or loss of health care coverage can seriously limit the job mobility of a worker. A worker changing from a large corporation to a small company could find his or her coverage reduced or even eliminated, and someone with a family member who has a preexisting condition might not be able to change jobs at all for fear of losing all coverage. Individually purchased insurance would eliminate that problem.

The more medical goods and services purchased directly by consumers, the greater the pressure exerted on providers to deliver high-quality care at reasonable prices. If consumers paid for most of their everyday expenses out of pocket and purchased insurance for catastrophic events, health insurance would function like other forms of insurance, such as automobile or homeowner's insurance. As a result the cost of such coverage would be considerably less.

A refundable tax credit could be offered to those whose income tax liability is less than the value of the credit. In that case the consumer would receive money back from the government, which would help to offset some of the payroll taxes paid by low-income families. Additional credits could be allowed for those whose medical bills exceed a certain amount of income during the year.[3]

[3]Several proposals offer tax credits for health care. For additional information, see Edmund F. Haislmaier, "Health Care for Workers and Their Families," in *Critical Issues: A National Health System for America*, ed. Stuart M. Butler and Edmund F. Haislmaier (Washington: Heritage Foundation, 1989), chap. 3, p. 59; Thomas H.

Making these changes in the tax code would allow the market to operate under less-hampered conditions. Consumers would react to prices, and their choices would force health care providers to adjust their offerings to meet the demand. The cost consciousness of consumers would have a dramatic impact on health care price inflation. In addition, the removal of a third party (the employer) from the equation would result in a reduction in paperwork and bureaucracy (currently a headache for both employer and employee) and would also diminish costs.

Objections to Changes in Tax Treatment

A number of objections have been raised to changing the status quo in the treatment of health care benefits. Among the most common are the following:

1. *People are used to receiving their health care benefits through their employer.* It is difficult for some people to imagine purchasing their own health insurance. Nevertheless, many Americans—including those who are self-employed, working for small businesses, and working part-time—are already paying for such insurance on their own. Traditionally, consumers have bought most of their own insurance, such as automobile and homeowner's insurance, and there really isn't any reason to treat health insurance differently.

2. *Elimination of the deduction for employer-provided coverage might encourage employers to eliminate other employee benefits.* Some workers and union officials have expressed concern that removing the tax incentives for employer-provided health coverage would lead to the elimination of other tax-free benefits. Workers must understand that the deduction or credit is not being eliminated; it is only being transferred from the employer directly to the employee. This arrangement would not affect other employee benefits.

3. *Insurance policies purchased by individuals would be more expensive than group insurance.* This objection is based on the premise that insurance companies incur higher costs in marketing policies and in making claims when they sell policies to individuals. Although that may be true in the theoretical sense, several changes actually would occur to lower costs.

Ainsworth, *Live or Die* (New York: Macmillan Publishing Company, 1983), pp. 96–100; and *An Agenda for Solving America's Health Care Crisis: A Task Force Report* (Dallas, 1990), pp. 11–15.

If consumers purchased policies that allowed for catastrophic coverage and paid for their everyday care out of pocket, those insurance policies would be much less expensive than policies that provide first-dollar coverage. Costs would be lower for health insurance companies because there would be fewer small claims and lower administrative costs for processing those claims.

Employees would still be able to obtain insurance through their companies by pooling their money through a voluntary payroll deduction. Allowing their employer to act as a broker in obtaining coverage would result in bulk savings that would be passed on to the individual employees.[4] Modifications could be made to the tax code to allow for the sale of group insurance through multiple employer trusts, trade groups and other nonprofit associations, and associations organized by employers.

If individual consumers purchased their own insurance, insurance companies would calculate premiums based on risk pools similar to the risk pools used to determine premiums for automobile, life, and homeowner's insurance. Currently, the risk pool used by an insurer usually consists of a single company. If one employee or a few employees in that company incur a significant health problem, premiums are likely to rise. That is especially true for smaller businesses, and occasionally a small company may find its insurance canceled because of employee illness. The risk pools under individually purchased insurance would be much larger, spreading the risk and reducing individual premiums. According to the 1990 Metropolitan Life survey (conducted by Louis Harris and Associates), 61 percent of the business, government, and health care leaders interviewed said they would accept paying health insurance premiums based on a community rate—rather than the experience of a single company.

Individuals faced with higher policy premiums because of high-risk situations or preexisting conditions could claim additional tax credits on their income tax to cover the higher premiums. The information supporting the additional credits could be verified by the insurance company.

4. *Consumers forced to pay for routine medical care would be discouraged from obtaining necessary care.* Allowing tax incentives for all individuals' health insurance premiums would

---

[4]See Haislmaier, pp. 63, 64.

increase access to medical care. In addition, such reforms would contribute to a reduction in the costs of health care, making it more affordable for consumers. First-dollar health coverage contributes to overuse, and increased consumer cost sharing does not lead to patient risk taking, such as sacrificing necessary health care.[5] There is no significant evidence that those who pay more out of pocket for routine expenses either delay treatment or do not seek necessary care.

5. *If the tax incentives for employer-provided coverage were eliminated, some individuals would not purchase their own insurance.* If tax incentives were offered to individuals, many previously uninsured people would have the opportunity to purchase insurance. The decline in the cost of coverage mentioned above would spur additional numbers of uninsured people to acquire coverage. A certain number who are willing to accept the risk may always remain uninsured by choice. There are other options for those who may still find coverage too costly, such as the very poor or those in high-risk categories (as discussed later in this chapter).

An added tax incentive could be given to individuals to help with out-of-pocket medical costs. This incentive would complement the purchase of health insurance covering catastrophic events. Individuals could make annual deposits to individual Medisave accounts (with a tax deduction or credit) and use the funds for routine medical expenses.[6] Medisave accounts would eliminate the need for individuals to purchase expensive first-dollar coverage, would give individuals control over their health care dollars, and would accumulate over time, allowing for lifetime and retirement health care planning. (In 1984 Singapore introduced a program under which all workers are required to contribute 6

[5]For an in-depth look at studies involving cost sharing, see R. Burciaga Valdez et al., "Consequences of Cost-Sharing for Children's Health," *Pediatrics* (May 1985): 952–61; and Kevin F. O'Grady et al., "The Impact of Cost-Sharing on Emergency Department Use," *New England Journal of Medicine* 313, no. 8 (August 22, 1985): 484–90.

[6]For a more complete discussion of the Medisave account, see National Center for Policy Analysis, pp. 16–18; John C. Goodman, Peter J. Ferrara, Gerald Musgrave, and Richard Rahn, *Solving the Problem of Medicare*, NCPA Policy Report no. 109 (Dallas: National Center for Policy Analysis, January 1984); and John C. Goodman and Richard Rahn, "Salvaging Medicare with an IRA," *Wall Street Journal*, March 20, 1984.

percent of their salaries to individual Medisave accounts. This program has eliminated the need for most third-party health insurance.)[7]

Reforms Benefiting Future Retirees and the Elderly

Improvements that would benefit the health care of future retirees and the current elderly population would expand individual choice and decrease use of and reliance on government programs. Permitting today's workers to prepare for their retirement so that they may be self-sufficient and purchase their own health care services would go a long way toward reducing the numbers of those who must rely on government for their health care needs.

Tax credits for the individual purchase of health insurance could also be claimed for money spent on the medical expenses of elderly relatives without the filer's having to meet the dependent support test. Current law mandates that, to claim a personal exemption, deduction, or credit, a taxpayer must demonstrate that he or she provided at least 50 percent of the dependent's total annual support. If that support test were eliminated or reduced, taxpayers could claim deductions or credits for money spent on the health care of relatives carried as dependents on their health insurance policies. That arrangement would encourage families to assume more responsibility for the health care of elderly relatives, thereby easing pressure on government programs.[8]

Some modifications of current law would help encourage the purchase of long-term care insurance. Insurance companies currently offer long-term care plans in several states, and the federal government has already taken a first step by applying to long-term care policies the same favorable tax treatment it applies to life insurance. Additional steps to be taken involve (1) allowing long-term care expenses to be eligible for the same tax credit as medical costs, (2) incorporating long-term care insurance into cafeteria employee benefit plans, (3) making modifications to allow workers to use their retirement funds to purchase long-term care insurance,

---

[7]For a discussion of Medisave accounts in Singapore, see John C. Goodman and Peter J. Ferrara, *Private Alternatives to Social Security in Other Countries*, NCPA Policy Report no. 132 (Dallas: National Center for Policy Analysis, April 1988).

[8]Haislmaier, p. 60.

(4) modifying life insurance policies to allow conversion into long-term care insurance policies, and (5) encouraging the development of financial instruments to enable the elderly to use the equity in their home to finance long-term care insurance or services.[9]

Another option, which has been introduced in Congress, is the health care savings account (HCSA) or medical IRA (MIRA). With an account similar to an IRA, workers could save, tax-free, during their working years to defray out-of-pocket health care expenses during retirement. Such accounts could be allowed to supplement, and even substitute for, future Medicare benefits. Because both social security and Medicare are pay-as-you-go programs in which there are no current savings to meet future obligations, tomorrow's obligations will have to be met with higher taxes on workers or the programs will face insolvency. HCSAs would reduce the future tax burden on workers while providing funds for retirees to pay medical expenses. Furthermore, using HCSAs would lessen the financial pressure on government programs.[10]

Changes should be made in the Medicare program so that instead of paying for routine medical care for the elderly, it would cover catastrophic illness, which is the area of most concern to retirees. The first step in this process would be to repeal all Medicare taxes and premiums on the elderly.

Eliminating the taxes and premiums now paid by the elderly would result in a revenue loss for the Medicare program. The loss could be offset by adjusting coinsurance and deductibles to give retirees protection against major illnesses and catastrophes while requiring them to pay out of pocket for routine medical expenses. Such a restructuring would mean that retirees would pay routine expenses but would be compensated with significant tax relief. Instead of being taxed to pay for the care of other Medicare beneficiaries, they would pay their own daily medical costs. And paying for routine care themselves would give them an incentive to seek out the most cost-effective treatment.

---

[9]Peter J. Ferrara, "Health Care and the Elderly," in *Critical Issues*, chap. 4, pp. 81–84.

[10]For more information on HCSAs, see National Center for Policy Analysis, pp. 25–27; Ferrara, "Health Care and the Elderly," pp. 87–89; and Peter J. Ferrara, "Long-Term Care: Why a New Entitlement Program Would Be Wrong," Cato Institute Policy Analysis, no. 144, December 13, 1990.

This reform would provide the elderly with the Medicare coverage needed for catastrophic illness without increasing the federal budget deficit. The costs the Medicare program incurs in providing for routine health care would be significantly reduced. Any such cost reductions would be offset to a degree by providing the elderly with the catastrophic illness coverage they need. In reality, the proposed reform would change the function of Medicare to one associated with traditional insurance programs.

The elderly poor would still receive their health coverage under the Medicaid program, and the rest of the elderly population would choose between paying the deductibles and coinsurance or purchasing private insurance or coverage by a health maintenance organization (HMO) to cover routine expenses.

Another element of reform would be to provide Medicare beneficiaries with vouchers, which they could use to purchase private health insurance coverage or other health plans, thereby replacing the current system in which Medicare itself is the insurer. The vouchers could also be used to pay hospitals and physicians directly. Vouchers would allow freedom of choice, and—within limits—retirees could choose the package of benefits and costs that best suited them, rather than being forced into a single plan, as they are under Medicare.

If the private plan provided minimum benefits at a cost less than the voucher amount, the retiree could pocket the difference. Retirees could choose coverage with very high deductibles, leaving them responsible for out-of-pocket expenses, or they could pay higher premiums for more extensive coverage. Retirees could be allowed to deposit any savings in an HCSA or an MIRA to help offset their everyday medical expenses.

Vouchers would increase competition because competing plans would strive to keep down costs and to provide better benefits, service, and care. Retirees would have the incentive to shop for the best coverage at the lowest cost in order to retain any savings. These modifications in the behavior of both retirees and insurance companies would slow the rise in health care costs and lessen pressures on the Medicare program.[11]

[11]For a more in-depth discussion of vouchers, see Ainsworth, p. 100; Ferrara, "Health Care and the Elderly," pp. 85–87; and National Center for Policy Analysis, pp. 27–28.

Limitations on coverage would aid in the conversion of the Medicare program to a more traditional catastrophic illness coverage plan. For example, the voucher amount could be limited to the purchase of catastrophic illness coverage only, with retirees then taking the responsibility for paying for routine expenses themselves.

Vouchers could also be used in the Veterans' Administration and Indian Health Service programs, altering their roles as direct providers of health care. For example, each veteran would be given a voucher with which he or she would purchase health insurance coverage. As with the Medicare voucher, the veteran would be free to choose the type and amount of coverage needed and to pocket any savings. Veterans would use the services of any private physician or hospital or, if they purchased an HMO-type plan, would use the HMO's doctors and hospitals. Or they could choose to purchase only catastrophic illness coverage and pay for routine medical expenses out of pocket.

Repeal of Mandated Benefits and Other Regulatory Legislation

As discussed in previous chapters, state-mandated health insurance benefits imposed by state governments, as well as a whole host of other federal and state regulations, increase the cost of health insurance and, in effect, price many consumers out of the market. State-mandated benefits should be repealed to permit consumers to buy no-frills health policies if that is their choice. Individuals should be free to buy the health coverage that is best suited to their needs; they should not have their options limited by the government.

In some states, mandated-benefits laws cover everything from heart and liver transplants to hairpieces and marriage counseling. Several states, including Arizona, Hawaii, Pennsylvania, and Washington, now require social and financial impact statements before passage of any additional mandates. (Interestingly, since Washington State instituted its policy in 1983, no new mandates have been adopted by the state legislature.)

Some observers have suggested that the federal government override state policy by permitting insurers to sell federally qualified health insurance plans both to individuals and to groups. Such insurance plans would be free from state-mandated benefits, state premium taxes, and mandatory contributions to state risk pools.[12] If granted, the override would mean that affordable polices would be available to those currently priced out of the health insurance market. Rep. Rod Chandler (R-Wash.) has sponsored a proposal that would allow small companies to purchase insurance by eliminating the ability of states to mandate the kinds of health benefits they must provide.

The barrage of regulations enacted in the past few decades must be repealed if the rise in health care costs is to be stemmed. Regulatory legislation—that which has given us such things as diagnostic related groups, prospective payment systems, certificates of need, and professional standards review organizations—was passed for the express purpose of controlling runaway costs, but it actually exacerbated costs by increasing bureaucracy, paperwork, and staffing requirements. Market-oriented reforms would render such legislation obsolete.

State regulatory laws should also undergo changes. States should abolish restrictive laws on the practice of medicine, including those involving licensing and the use of paraprofessionals. Passed under the guise of protecting the consumer and supported by the medical associations, such laws have had the effect of keeping costs high. They shelter the economic interests of physicians by preserving the medical monopoly and restricting other professionals, such as nurses and physician's assistants, from performing certain routine procedures.[13] State licensing could be replaced by private organizations operating like a Better Business Bureau for physicians, which patients could call to obtain information about particular physicians.

Health Care for High-Risk Individuals, the Very Poor, and the Uninsured

The very poor, the uninsured, and those in high-risk categories of illness offer a challenge to people who devise market solutions to health coverage. Traditionally, those in high-risk categories of illness have had a more difficult time obtaining affordable health insurance. The very poor, on the other hand, usually receive their

---

[12]National Center for Policy Analysis, p. 20.

[13]The effect of regulatory and licensing procedures is discussed in more detail in Chapter 3, and in John C. Goodman, *The Regulation of Medical Care: Is the Price Too High?* (Washington: Cato Institute, 1980).

health care through a government agency or health center, but common complaints include inadequate treatment and low-quality care. Those who are uninsured remain so for a variety of reasons, but a significant number of them would probably prefer to have health insurance. The following section provides suggestions for reforms that would alleviate the problems facing these groups.

High-Risk Individuals

Why is it that some Americans have such difficulty obtaining health insurance? One reason is that in almost every state, health insurance premium prices are regulated. Regulation places a restriction on how much premium prices may increase to cover rising health care costs. Most states will not allow premium price increases unless the benefits paid are equal to at least a percentage of premium income. Essentially, the regulation of premium prices is the regulation of profits.

Without profits, insurance companies cannot build up the reserves they need to cover unusual costs, such as those associated with high-risk individuals. When an insurance company takes on a high-risk individual, it is taking on more financial risk. If the state government regulates the amount of profit a company can make, high-risk individuals will find themselves unable to obtain health insurance.

Once the state government has forced insurers out of the high-risk market, it must step in and provide the insurance, usually through a risk pool. Health insurance risk pools, like automobile insurance risk pools, are a mechanism for ensuring that insurance is available to high-risk people who are now considered uninsurable. Costs are borne entirely by those in the risk pool or are subsidized by government or by premiums of nonrisk-pool policies. Some state and federal organizations help reduce premiums by providing reinsurance for losses beyond a certain level. The reinsurance pool is essentially insurance for the risk pool, and it is funded by the state government or by assessments of insurance companies.

Fifteen states have enacted laws establishing health insurance risk pools.[14] States generally operate such pools by forming an

[14]Connecticut, Florida, Illinois, Indiana, Iowa, Maine, Minnesota, Montana, Nebraska, New Mexico, North Dakota, Oregon, Tennessee, Washington, and Wisconsin.

association of all health insurance companies doing business in the state. One insurance organization normally is selected to administer the plan under specific guidelines for benefits, premiums, and deductibles.

Insurance for high-risk individuals obviously is more expensive than that for standard-risk individuals. But in a risk pool, premiums are set at a level affordable by those enrolled in the pool, so the enrollees pay less in premiums than the cost of the services they use. Because all states cap the price of risk-pool insurance, risk pools almost always lose money. The most common approach to covering the losses incurred by a pool is to require insurance companies to contribute in proportion to their share of the state health insurance market. Some states partly offset this assessment through some form of tax credit against premium taxes or other state taxes.

Federal legislation to encourage all states to set up risk pools has been considered recently. Under one proposal, federal assistance would be provided for states to use either to establish risk pools or, for those with existing pools, to improve access to affordable insurance. Another proposal would mandate participation in an established risk pool by all employers doing business in a state.

The major problem with risk pools is that they raise the cost of health care for everyone. Taxes levied on hospital revenues, assessments on insurers, and even credits allowed against other state taxes all generate pressures to increase costs or taxes, or both. The existence of risk pools may encourage insurers to become more selective in issuing individual policies, forcing more individuals who are less healthy into risk pools to obtain coverage. The additional pressure on state governments to subsidize the risk pools is burdensome, as most are already struggling with budget deficits.

A market-oriented alternative to state-mandated risk pools would be to allow insurers on their own, or in combination with other insurers, to provide federally qualified high-risk insurance. Such insurance plans would offer catastrophic illness insurance policies only. Individuals who purchased high-risk insurance would be permitted federal income tax deductions of up to twice an amount of premium adjusted for age and family size.[15]

---

[15]See John C. Goodman, *Mandating Health Insurance*, NCPA Policy Report no. 136 (Dallas: National Center for Policy Analysis, February 1989), pp. 20–21.

Some Blue Cross and Blue Shield plans operate as de facto high-risk pools in a number of states by providing open-enrollment periods during which any group can buy insurance.[16] Of the 74 Blue Cross and Blue Shield organizations nationwide, 21 offer open enrollment. Open-enrollment plans offer coverage at substantially lower cost than the rates charged by state pools. Employers who buy open-enrollment plans are insulated from the premium spikes they can experience with other insurers once someone in the group becomes very ill. Such plans use community rating to calculate premium increases. All companies buying one of these policies are in the same risk pool, and all pay the same rates.

Enacting market reforms and reducing government regulations will lower the cost of health care in general, making insurance for high-risk individuals easier to obtain. Offering a tax credit for the individual purchase of health insurance will allow workers to retain the same policy when they switch or lose their jobs, effectively eliminating many of the problems associated with a medically high-risk individual who seeks new coverage. Offering additional tax credits or a refundable tax credit to those with proportionally higher medical expenses would provide added tax relief for high-risk consumers.

Low-Income People and the Very Poor

Breaking the health care cost spiral by implementing market-based reforms will provide the greatest assistance to those with low incomes. As health care costs fall, health insurance will become more affordable. The pressure on government programs for health care will lessen as more of the uninsured poor are able to obtain health care coverage on their own. Removing federal and state regulations, like removing mandated-benefits laws, would make it possible for low-income consumers to purchase less-expensive, no-frills insurance for catastrophic illness.

Additional changes could be made in the health care system to assist low-income people. Those who have no tax liability could be provided with a refundable tax credit to aid them in purchasing health care coverage. The credit would be equal to a percentage of

[16]Open-enrollment plans operate in Alabama, the District of Columbia, Maryland, Massachusetts, Michigan, New Hampshire, New Jersey, New York, North Carolina, Pennsylvania, Rhode Island, Vermont, and Virginia.

premium costs and would be phased out as income surpassed the poverty level. In effect, the credit would be a voucher for low-income citizens to use in buying health insurance. Sen. Lloyd Bentsen (D-Tex.) has proposed legislation that includes refundable tax credits for the purchase of health insurance.

To aid families that have needy relatives, taxpayers could take tax credits for money spent on the medical expenses of their relatives without having to meet the dependent support test. This proposal is similar to the tax credit for taxpayers providing health care for elderly relatives (covered earlier in this chapter).

For the very poor, who may remain within a government health program, the objective would be to keep program operations at the level closest to the recipient—preferably the state or local level. At those levels the poor would receive more individualized attention, and there would be less bureaucracy. The federal government should give states more flexibility in designing their Medicaid and other health programs for the poor. Reducing the amount of regulation, along with allowing for modifications in state programs to meet different needs, would improve services for the poor while contributing to cost containment. Examples incorporating this kind of flexibility are some of the health care demonstration projects currently operating in several states.[17] The federal government should continue to give states this kind of adaptability so as to provide the very poor with more personalized service at lower costs to the taxpayer.

Another option for the very poor would be to give Medicaid recipients a voucher with which they could purchase their medical care. They would be given an amount based on family size and income and would be free to purchase health insurance or to enroll in an HMO or a managed-care plan. Although they would be required to show that they did purchase some kind of health coverage, they could pocket any left-over money. This arrangement would encourage recipients to shop around for the best coverage at the lowest price.

[17]For more information on such demonstration projects, see Terree P. Wasley, "Health Care for the Poor, Unemployed, and High-Risk," in *Critical Issues*, chap. 5, pp. 98–108.

In addition, states could use refundable deductibles in capitation plans for the poor.[18] Under a refundable-deductible system, a state could enroll beneficiaries in a capitation plan that includes deductibles similar to those used in normal insurance. The difference would be that the state would prepay the deductible and then refund any unused portion to the beneficiary at the end of the year. In this way the poor would have an incentive to avoid unnecessary or costly care.

Such an incentive is important because Medicaid patients tend to use costly and inappropriate care, such as making unnecessary visits to hospital emergency rooms rather than seeing a family doctor. This practice has added considerably to Medicaid budgets in the past, and some observers have suggested that Medicaid patients be charged deductibles and copayments. However, the difficulty with this proposal is that the very poor often cannot afford the copayments and deductibles. Under plans with refundable deductibles, patients' medical care is paid for, but they still have some incentive to seek the most cost-effective treatment because they will receive any savings at the end of the year. Such a system could significantly reduce overuse and excessive treatment, thereby reducing program costs and making more efficient use of every dollar spent.

One of the traditional methods of providing medical care for the poor must not be forgotten in the rush to provide new programs. Most people assume that, although physicians once treated poor patients for free, they cannot or will not assume that responsibility anymore. However, most physicians indicate that they do not charge patients who cannot afford to pay. As mentioned in Chapter 2, physicians provided uncompensated care that amounted to $10.2 billion in 1989, and the proportion of physicians providing charity care rose to 66 percent in 1989 from 62 percent in 1988.[19] One doctor I spoke with said she requires all her patients to pay something,

[18]An HMO is an example of a capitation plan, in which the HMO contracts with a medical practice and caps payments for services.

[19]From the AMA's Socioeconomic Monitoring System 1990 core and autumn surveys, provided in correspondence from Lynn Jensen of the AMA, and from the 1989 Physician Masterfile, *Physician Characteristics and Distribution* (Chicago: AMA, Department of Physician Data Services, Division of Survey and Data Resources, 1990).

146

even if it is only one dollar, and she also accepts barter payment—and has accepted such payment in the form of dill pickles and homemade jelly.

The Uninsured

Although there are individuals who have freely chosen to remain uninsured, many people do find the purchase of insurance out of their reach. Many of these uninsured are owners of small businesses and their employees, the self-employed, and part-time workers. Reduced health care costs would solve the problem of unaffordable health insurance for a lot of them.

Providing an individual tax credit for the purchase of health coverage would allow many currently uninsured people to obtain insurance. Repealing many of the regulatory laws, such as those mandating benefits, would allow the uninsured to purchase no-frills coverage for catastrophic illness that would protect them against overwhelming medical expenses.

An estimated two-thirds of small businesses nationwide offer health coverage.[20] But more than one-half of uninsured working individuals are employed by firms with 25 or fewer employees.[21] According to a survey made early in 1991 by National Small Business United, a Washington-based group, insurance rates had increased between 16 and 35 percent since 1990 for 38 percent of the business owners polled.[22]

Some states have already revised their mandated-benefits laws to allow companies to offer bare-bones health plans. In Florida, Virginia, and Washington, new laws permit experimental, limited coverage for small companies that don't already offer health benefits. In Connecticut a recently passed law temporarily reduces rates for small firms and establishes a pooling arrangement to cover people with existing medical conditions. Blue Cross companies in Oklahoma and California recently started offering lower-cost, bare-bones insurance policies to small groups. The state governments of

[20]Employee Benefit Research Institute, "Features of Employer-Sponsored Health Plans," *Issue Brief* no. 100, Washington, March 1990.

[21]Pamela Farley Short, Alan C. Monheit, and Karen Beauregard, *A Profile of Uninsured Americans* (Washington: Department of Health and Human Services, DHHS Publication no. 89-3443, September 1989), p. 13.

[22]Small Business USA, "Member Survey Results: Access to Health Care" (Washington: National Small Business United, May/June 1990), p. 7.

Indiana, Nebraska, and even Massachusetts are considering similar programs.

Multiple employer trusts (METs), which have been developed in various parts of the country in recent years, enable self-employed workers and small business owners with very limited or no insurance plans to purchase more comprehensive, affordable coverage on a pooled basis.

Many small businesses are able to purchase health coverage through a business group or coalition. In Cleveland, Ohio, for example, the Council of Smaller Enterprises, a division of the Greater Cleveland Growth Association (the chamber of commerce) manages a wide range of services for member companies, including employee benefit programs.[23] The Council oversees a $140 million investment in health care for over 130,000 residents and offers its members health care coverage. Because it can pool a number of small businesses into a larger group, it is able to offer health insurance at more affordable rates.

Other examples are the Small Business Service Bureau, a Massachusetts-based association that arranges group insurance through HMOs and Blue Cross organizations for 35,000 small businesses across the country; the New Castle County Chamber of Commerce in Newark, Delaware, which manages a group-purchasing arrangement for small employers in the area; and the Chamber of Commerce in San Francisco, which recently launched a group-purchasing arrangement.

Many states are offering low-cost pilot projects that help small businesses purchase health insurance. The projects are designed to attract small, uninsured companies. For example, the Health Care Group of Arizona, which is contained within the state's alternative to the Medicaid program and is called the Arizona Health Care Cost Containment System (AHCCCS), offers coverage to the working uninsured.[24] The state administers the program through the AHCCCS, and premiums are around 30 percent less for those

[23]Council of Smaller Enterprises, *Employee Benefits Program 1990–91* (Cleveland: Greater Cleveland Growth Association, 1990).

[24]Jack Meyer, Sean Sullivan, and Sharon Silow-Carroll, "Private Sector Initiatives: Controlling Health Care Costs," a report by New Directions for Policy to the Federation of American Health Systems (Washington: Health Leadership Council, March 1991), p. 43.

seeking coverage. Companies can participate if they have 25 or fewer employees and haven't offered them health insurance during the past six months. The employer decides which plan to offer and may or may not help pay the premiums. The plan, currently financed by grants from private entities, is eventually expected to become self-supporting.

In Denver, the Shared Cost Option for Private Employers (SCOPE) accepts small companies seeking to switch to less-expensive health plans, as well as those currently uninsured. SCOPE provides health insurance for 611 companies covering 5,500 individuals.[25] It also operates without a government subsidy and cuts premium costs by requiring relatively high deductibles and coinsurance.

Other states, such as Maine, Michigan, Tennessee, Utah, and Wisconsin, are offering plans for bare-bones insurance coverage for the uninsured at a reduced cost. In 1990 the state of Oregon began to offer tax credits to small businesses that provide health coverage for employees. Companies with 25 or fewer employees that participate in the program receive a monthly credit of $25 per worker.

The Pioneer Institute for Public Policy Research in Boston is promoting an alternative to the Massachusetts Health Plan for the uninsured. Instead of the mandatory employer-supplied health insurance plan, the institute has recommended a tax credit for health care services.[26] Under the plan, every resident of Massachusetts who is without health insurance coverage and who is not eligible for coverage under a public or a private health insurance plan would receive a state income tax credit equal to a percentage of the average health insurance premium. The percentage would depend on the level of family income and the size of the family.

The tax credit received by a family would have to be applied toward the purchase of an insurance policy or a prepaid plan (such as an HMO) of the individual's choice. The tax credit would be less than the expected insurance premium, so that recipients would have a strong incentive to shop around for the least expensive coverage to minimize their own share of the premium costs. Unlike

[25]Ibid., p. 41.

[26]Altiat F. Ott and Wayne B. Gray, *The Massachusetts Health Plan: The Right Prescription?* (Boston: Pioneer Institute for Public Policy Research, 1988).

the mandatory employer-supplied plans currently in effect in Massachusetts, this plan would enhance the ability of families to purchase health insurance, and it would enhance individual choice.[27]

Conclusion

There are those who say that we've tried a free market for our health care and it just hasn't worked; our only alternative is to adopt a national health insurance plan so that everyone will have access to health care. But the historical examination undertaken in this book reveals that a market in health care has never truly existed in the United States. The development of the U.S. health care system has been riddled with government interference, regulation, and protection, often with the encouragement and support of business, industry, and medical associations.

In our haste to adopt what to some seems like the only solution left, we should look carefully at the experience of other countries. We are at a crossroads in world history: socialism and communism have been repudiated as viable economic systems, and countries everywhere are embracing market systems and the freedom of individuals to make their own choices. If nation after nation has realized that collectivism and nationalization do not work, on either a national or an individual level, then why would anyone expect nationalization to be a success in a specific area, such as health care? An examination of the Canadian, British, and other national health care systems reveals their inferiority—they provide a much lower quality of care overall, with high costs and oppressive limits on freedom of choice. The nationalization of health care removes the freedom of choice and lowers the quality of life and care for both patients and physicians, leaving an impersonal government bureaucracy to decide who will live and who will die.

Although the proposed solutions are varied, it has become clear to all that the American system of health care is in need of comprehensive reform. Some people, without taking heed of the rejection of nationalized systems worldwide and the dismal record of national health care in other countries, would offer a nationalized system as the only solution to problems of access and cost.

---

[27]For more information on the tax credit, see Ott and Gray, pp. 99–110.

150

People, not just in the United States but all over the world, want freedom of choice. And they want it in all areas of their lives. The watchword for American consumers of health care services should be "choice"—allowing people to choose their health care and coverage from a wide array of options. The recommendations in this book would go a long way toward designing a health care system that would be based on the market. Such a system would offer maximum freedom of choice and provide sufficient coverage and quality care at costs all our citizens could afford.

Index

AALL. *See* American Association of
  Labor Legislation (AALL)
AAPS News, 2n2, 24n74, 28n79
AAPS survey (Association of American
  Physicians and Surgeons survey),
  24, 26, 27, 28
Abramowitz, Kenneth, 13
Act for Relief of Sick and Disabled
  Seamen (1799), 38
Adams, John, 38
AFL-CIO national health insurance
  campaign, 82–83
AHA. *See* American Hospital
  Association (AHA)
Ainsworth, Thomas H., 41, 134n3,
  139n11
Alcohol, Drug Abuse, and Mental
  Health Block Grant program, 65–66
Allen, Ernest M., 59n40
Alper, Philip R., 25n76
AMA. *See* American Medical
  Association (AMA)
AMA Gallup poll (1991), 15
AMA opinion surveys (1990), 11, 12,
  13–14, 28n80
American Academy of Family
  Physicians, 85
American Association of Labor
  Legislation (AALL), 78
American Association of Retired
  Persons (AARP), 85–86
American College of Healthcare
  Executives, 102
American College of Physicians (ACP),
  7n12, 85, 121–22
American Healthcare Systems
  Institute, 23
American Hospital Association (AHA),
  34–35, 60
American Medical Association (AMA),
  6n6, 17n49
  antitrust violation by, 53
  Council on Medical Education, 41,
    43, 44
  dissent to, 79–80

establishment of (1847), 40–41
opposition to lodge practice and
  company doctors, 45–47
opposition to prepaid plans and
  medical cooperatives, 52
position on health insurance bill
  (1906), 78
position on proposed group practice
  and payment, 79
power of, 41–44, 46–47
support for licensing laws by, 41–42
use of Flexner Report by, 43–44
AmeriCare proposal, 119–21, 127
Anavy, Daniel, 94n38
Anderson, Kevin, 15n43
Anderson, Odin W., 56n37
Anderson, William, 26
Arizona
  Gallup poll (1991), 6
  Health Care Cost Containment
    System (AHCCCS), 148–49
Association of American Physicians
  and Surgeons survey (1990), 127
Austria, 77

Bacon, Kenneth H., 17n48, 68n69,
  84nn12, 13, 86n19, 126
Baker, Charles D., 113nn106, 107, 108
Balance billing, 25–26
Barnes, John A., 96n48, 97n50
Baylor University Hospital, 48, 52
  See also Multiple-hospital insurance
    plans
Beauregard, Karen, 147n21
Benefits societies, 46–47
Berman, Howard J., 50
Berry, Cindi, 66n55
Billett, Michael, 96, 99
Bismarck, Otto von, 88
Blendon, Robert, 14, 15nn41, 44
Block grant programs, 65–66
Blue Cross/Blue Shield Gallup poll
  (1990), 14

Council of Smaller Enterprises, Ohio, 148
Coutts, Jane, 101n65
Crane, Mark, 6n8
Crenshaw, Albert B., 84nn11, 14
Crosby, John B., 102

Davis, Karen, 61nn45, 46
Deets, Horace, 86
Defensive medicine, 12
Denmark, 77, 92
Diagnostic related groups (DRGs), 34, 72
Dickson, Thomas, 95
Donelan, Karen, 15n44
Donnelly, Brian, 34, 126
Dukakis, Michael, 111

Elderly people
    See also Medicaid program; Medicare program
    effect of increased insurance costs on, 69
    government health care programs for, 61–62
Ellwood, Paul, 69–70
Employee Benefit Research Institute, 147n20
Employers
    See also Company doctors
    cost-control measures of, 74–75
    early health insurance plans of, 45
    health insurance plans of, 55–57
    increase in premiums for, 67–68
Endicott, Kenneth M., 59n40
European Community, 92
European governments, 77, 87–92
    See also specific countries

Farmers Union Hospital Association, 52
Feder, Don, 94nn39, 40, 42
Feldman, Jacob J., 56n37
Ferrara, Peter J., 136n6, 137n7, 138nn9, 10, 139n11
Ferrier, Ian, 100n64
Filak, Michael, 19–20
Finkelstein, James, 108
Flexner, Abraham, 42–43
Flexner, Simon, 43

Flexner Report (1910), 42–44
Florida, 147
Food, Drug, and Cosmetic Act (1962 amendments), 74
Food and Drug Administration (FDA), 74
Ford Motor Company, 57
Forgotson, Edward H., 42n7
Fortune poll (1991), 6, 12–13
France, 77
Fraternal orders, 45, 46–47
Frazier, Irene, 34
Freedom of choice
    See also Responsibility, individual
    as alternative to national health care, 127–28
    demand for, 151
    nationalized health care eliminates, 150
    proposed mechanism to encourage, 132–34
    reforms to make transition to, 129–32
Free-market system
    reforms to make transition to, 129–32
    role of comparable worth concept in, 124–25

Gallup poll (1990), 6
Garbarino, Joseph W., 56n36
Garfield, Sidney, 52
Gausewitz, Phillips, 74n81
General Motors, 57
Germany, 77, 88–89, 91
Glanville, Paul, 2, 18–19
Globerman, Steven, 95n44
Goldberg, Jacob A., 43n10
Gompers, Samuel, 78
Goodman, John C., 41n5, 43n10, 51n26, 67, 71n73, 73n79, 99nn58, 59, 115n109, 116, 136n6, 137n7, 141n13, 143n15
Goodman, William E., 98, 106–7
Government role
    See also Health insurance; Health care system, national; Legislation; Regulation
    in expansion in health care arena, 53–54, 57, 59–66
    in experience rating, 58
    in financing and regulation of HMOs, 70, 123

as response to rising health care costs, 69–70, 81–82
as source of rising health care costs, 19–21
use of capitation plan by, 146n18
Health Professions Education Assistance Act (1963), 61
Health programs, government
    See also Indian Health Service; Medicaid; Medicare; U. S. Department of Defense (DoD) health care system; Veterans' Administration medical services
    expansion of federal, 59
    Medicare and Medicaid, 61
    for unemployed, poor, and elderly, 61
Health Security Plan (1970), 81
Heartbeat Windsor, 96, 99
Hershey, Stephen, 13, 18
Herzlinger, Regina E., 67nn64, 65
HIAA. See Health Insurance Association of America (HIAA)
Higgins (A. Foster) and Company survey, 9
Hill-Burton Act. See Hospital Survey and Construction Act (Hill-Burton Act, 1946)
HMOs. See Health maintenance organizations (HMOs)
Holzman, David, 66n56
Hoover, Herbert, 39
Hospital associations, 46
    See also Insurance companies
Hospitals
    administered by Veterans' Administration, 60
    anti-competitive activities of, 47
    of Departments of Defense and Veterans' Affairs, 65
    effect of construction regulation on, 33–34
    effect of government intervention on, 30–31, 60
    effect of health care costs on, 30
    effect of Medicare and Medicaid programs on, 63–64
    financing of Canadian, 93
    incentives to provide treatment, 57–58
    increased number of, 45
    insurance reimbursement problems of, 32–33
    ownership by government, Great Britain, 87

reimbursed by cost-plus method, 50–51
    uncompensated care provided by, 32
Hospital Survey and Construction Act (Hill-Burton Act, 1946), 33, 60, 64
Howard, James S., 84n15
Hoye, Lorna, 95n44
Hudson, Alan R., 13
Hungary, 77

Income redistribution, 104
Indiana, 148
Indian Health Service, 64–65
Inland Steel case (1949), 56
Insurance
    long-term care, 137–38
    malpractice/liability, 22–24, 68–69, 112
Insurance companies
    See also Blue Cross; Blue Shield; Reinsurance pools; Risk pool insurance
    effect of premium regulation on, 142
    health plans of, 49
    influence of first-dollar coverage on, 58
Ireland, 92
Italy, 77

Jackson, Estele, 14n38, 15n42
Jensen, Lynn, 14n36
Johnson, Lyndon B., 40

Kaiser Industries, 52
Karr, Albert R., 84n10
Kelly, John T., 21
Kennedy, Edward M., 81, 82, 115, 119
Kennedy bill. See Minimum Health Benefits for All Workers Act (S.768 and H.R.1845)
Kerr-Mills legislation (1960), 61
Kessel, Reuben A., 43nn9, 10, 44
Kilpatrick, Lynne, 125n120, 126n121
Koch, John, 11, 21
Krasny, Jacques, 100n64

Labor unions
    AFL-CIO national health insurance campaign, 82–83

157

establishment (1965), 62, 81
fixed fee schedule under, 72–73
problems of bureaucracy in, 24–28
proposed changes for catastrophic
  health care under, 138–40
proposed changes in, 138–40
proposed voucher system under,
  139
recommended changes in, 138
reimbursement problems of, 34–35
spending under, 66
Medisave accounts, 136–37
  See also Medical IRA (MIRA)
Mental health research, 59
Metropolitan Life survey (1990), 11,
  16, 83n8, 115
Meyer, Jack, 9nn18, 20, 66n57, 69n71,
  148n24, 149n25
Michigan, 149
Michigan Hospital Association, 34
Minimum Health Benefits for All
  Workers Act (S.768 and H.R.1845),
  115–17, 120, 127
MIRA. *See* Medical IRA (MIRA)
Mises, Ludwig von, 128
Mitchell, George, 119
Mobley, Michael, 22
Modern Healthcare survey, 3
Monheit, Alan C., 147n21
Multiple employer trusts (METs), 148
Multiple-hospital insurance plans,
  48–49
Musgrave, Gerald L., 51n26, 73n79,
  136n6

Nabil, Sheila, 18, 19
NAM. *See* National Association of
  Manufacturers (NAM)
National Academy of Sciences, 37
National Association of Manufacturers
  (NAM), 78
National Center for Policy Analysis,
  51–52n26, 67nn61, 62, 63, 73nn77,
  78, 103–4, 136n6, 139n11
National Federation of Independent
  Business survey (1989), 9, 85
National Health Interview Survey
  (1984), 112
National Health Planning and
  Resources Development Act (1974),
  71
National Health Service, Great Britain,
  87–88, 89–91

National Heart Institute, 59
National Institute of Mental Health
  (NIMH), 59–60
National Institutes of Health (NIH)
  legislated role of, 53–54
  post–World War II expansion, 59
National Leadership Coalition for
  Health Care Reform, 83
National Quarantine Services Act
  (1878), 37
National Science Foundation, 59
National Small Business United survey
  (1991), 10, 147
Nation's Business health care survey
  (1990), 9
Nebraska, 148
Nelson, Charles, 7n11
Netherlands, the, 77, 89, 92
Neuhauser, Duncan, 45n15
Neuschler, Edward, 99n60, 100, 103
New Castle County Chamber of
  Commerce, 148
New Deal, 38, 40
Newfoundland Medical Association,
  101
Newman, Roger, 42n7
New York Ophthalmology Society v.
  Bowen, 25
NIH. *See* National Institutes of Health
  (NIH)
Nixon, Richard M., 82
Norway, 77
Novack, Jane, 108nn91, 92
Nowotny, Otto H., 131

O'Grady, Kevin F., 136n5
Oklahoma, 147
Ontario Pay Equity Commission,
  125–26
Oregon, 149
Oregon Basic Health Services Act
  (1989), 109–10
Orndorff, Beverly, 14n38, 15n42
Osler, William, 40
Ott, Attiat F., 111–12, 149n26, 150n27

Parlett, Don, 13
Parran, Thomas, 54
Parsons, Paul, 12, 21, 22, 29
Pasteur, Louis, 40
Pay equity. *See* Comparable worth
  concept

159

Pepper, Claude, 117
Pepper Commission. *See* U. S.
    Bipartisan Commission on
    Comprehensive Health Care (Pepper
    Commission)
Physicians
    See also Company doctors; Defensive
        medicine; Lodge practice
    administrative costs of, 17–19
    changing role in early 1900s of, 40
    early retirement decision by, 28–29
    effect of Medicare and Medicaid
        programs on, 63–64
    effect of proposed Pepper
        Commission legislation on, 118–19
    government role to increase supply,
        61
    impact of Flexner Report on
        minority, 43–44
    impact of licensing laws on, 41–42
    incentives to provide treatment,
        57–58
    legislation restricting, 69–73
    licensing of, 41–42
    problems with Medicare
        bureaucracy, 24–28
    reimbursement by cost-plus method,
        51
    response to proposed Medicare
        changes, 127
    uncompensated care by, 13–14, 146
Physicians for a National Health
    Program (PNHP), 85, 104–5
Physician viewpoint
    on early retirement, 28
    on Medicare program, 24–28
    of physician-patient relationship,
        19–21
    in relations with AMA, 41
Pioneer Institute for Public Policy
    Research, 149
PNHP. *See* Physicians for a National
    Health Program (PNHP)
Poor people
    See also Medicaid program
    access to health care by, 13–14
    effect of increased insurance costs
        on, 69
    health care system changes to assist,
        145–46
    increased access to health care for,
        61–62
PPOs. *See* Preferred provider
    organizations (PPOs)

Preferred provider organizations
    (PPOs), 2
Premiums
    calculation of, 58
    community rating and experience
        rating to calculate, 58
    increase in, 67–68
    for liability insurance, 23
    for malpractice insurance, 69
    under Medicaid and Medicare, 63
    proposed tax credits for, 132
    recommended repeal of elderly
        Medicare, 138
    in risk pools, 143
    state regulation of, 142
Prepaid health plans
    emergence of, 46–47, 52–53
    of hospital associations, 46
    medical societies' role in regulation
        of, 53
Preventive Health and Health Services
    Block Grant program, 65
Professional standards review
    organizations (PSROs), 71
Prospective payment system (PPS),
    72–73
Pryor, David, 127
PSROs. *See* Professional standards
    review organizations (PSROs)
Public health services, U.S., 37–39, 54
Public Law 89–290 (1964), 61
Puccini, Art, 84
Pure Food and Drug Act, 38

Rachlis, Michael, 101
Rahn, Richard, 136n6
Rand, Ayn, 37
Ransdell Act (1930), 53–54
Rayack, Elton, 44n12
RBRVS. *See* Resource-based relative-
    value scale (RBRVS)
Reagan, Ronald, 82
Regulation
    See also Licensing laws
    cost of, 30–33
    effect on costs, 74
    exemption from, 49–50
    has increased government control,
        123
    of HMOs, 70, 123
    of hospital construction, 33–34, 60
    medical societies as force for, 53
    of premiums, 142

related to Medicare reimbursement, 63–64

resource-based relative-value scale (RBRVS) under, 123–24

Reigle, Donald, 119

Reimbursement
cost-plus under Blue Cross (1930s), 50–51
hospital problems with, 34–35
Medicare and Medicaid cost-plus system of, 63
physician problems with, 26–27
under prospective payment system, 72–73

Reinhardt, Uwe E., 90

Reinsurance pools, 142
See also Risk pool insurance

Relman, Arnold, 85

Resettlement Administration, 79

Resource-based relative-value scale (RBRVS), 123–27

Responsibility, individual, 130–32
See also Freedom of choice

Reuther, Walter, 81

Ricardo-Campbell, Rita, 130n1

Richmond, Isabelle, 91–92

Ricklefs, Roger, 8n15, 9nn16, 20, 85n16

Risk pool insurance, 142–43

Robbins, Aldona, 104, 106, 115n109, 116

Robbins, Gary, 104, 106, 115n109, 116

Rockefeller, Jay, 118n112, 119

Rockefeller Institute for Medical Research, 43

Roemer, Ruth, 42n7

Roentgen, Wilhelm, 40

Roosevelt, Franklin D., 38, 40, 54, 79

Roosevelt, Theodore, 37

Roseboom, Eugene H., 80n5

Rosenblatt, Cheryl, 20

Ross-Loos Clinic, 52

Ruffenach, Glenn, 21n62, 85n17

Rundle, Rhonda L., 33n94

Russia, 77

San Francisco Chamber of Commerce, 148

Schildt, Annika, 91nn32, 33

Schoen, Cathy, 61nn45, 46

Schramm, Carl J., 5n2, 6n4, 7

Schwartz, Jeffrey, 67nn64, 65

SCOPE. See Shared Cost Option for Private Employers (SCOPE), Denver

Scully, Tom, 120

Serbia, 77

Shadid, Michael, 52–53

Shared Cost Option for Private Employers (SCOPE), Denver, 149

Sheeline, William E., 6n7

Sheppard-Towner Act, 38

Sherman Antitrust Act, 53

Short, Kathleen, 7n11

Short, Pamela Farley, 147n21

Shyrock, Richard H., 43n10

Silow-Carroll, Sharon, 3n3, 9nn18, 20, 66n57, 69n71, 148n24, 149n25

Small business
effect of experience rating on, 58
effect of high insurance rates on, 147
effect of increased premiums on, 67–68
insurance rates for, 9–10
mechanisms for purchase of health insurance, 148

Small Business Service Bureau, 148

Small Business USA, 9n17

Smith, Lee, 10n23, 12n27, 13n33, 92n34, 94n37

Societies
benefits, 46–47
medical, 41–42, 47, 52–53

Sodaro, Edward R., 24

Solon, E. M., 23nn69, 70

Specter, Michael, 92n35, 95nn45, 46, 97n52

Spending, health care, 2–3
Canadian and U.S., 99–100
increase in hospital, 63
Medicaid and Medicare, 66
personal, 66–67

Stark, Pete, 34, 115, 127

Starr, Paul, 38n2, 39n3, 46nn16, 17, 47n18, 52nn27, 28, 29, 54n31, 55n32, 59nn38, 39, 42, 78nn1, 2, 80nn3, 4, 82nn6, 7

Stearn, Martha, 24, 26–27

Steinfeld, Jesse L., 54n30

Steinwald, Bruce, 45n15

Stephens, Michael D., 33

Stevens, Carol, 14n39

Stout, Hilary, 68n67

Sullivan, Sean, 9nn18, 20, 66n57, 69n71, 148n24, 149n25

Sundwall, David, 23

Sweden, 77, 88, 91

Switzerland, 77

Swoboda, Frank, 83n9, 84nn11, 14

161

Taxation
  Blue Cross exemption from, 49–50
  of first-dollar health insurance, 57
  objections to changes in, 134–37
  recommended repeal of elderly
    Medicare, 138
Tax credit
  conditions for refund, 133
  for covering risk pool losses, 143–44
  effect of proposed, 147
  proposal to establish system for,
    132–33, 137
  proposed for uninsured in
    Massachusetts, 149–50
Tennessee, 149
Thomas, Lewis, 40n4
Thompson, Roger, 9n19, 16n47
Time/CNN poll (1991), 5, 7n10, 14
Todd, James, 17
Toronto Board of Health, 101
Toth, John, 12
Truman, Harry S, 80, 81

Uncompensated care, 13–14, 32, 146
Uninsured people
  characteristics of, 147
  incidence in U.S. of, 111–12
  state-mandated programs for,
    109–15
  state-offered health insurance for,
    149
  tax credit in Massachusetts for, 149
United Automobile Workers (UAW),
  57
U.S. Bipartisan Commission on
  Comprehensive Health Care (Pepper
  Commission), 117–19
  See also AmeriCare proposal
U.S. Bureau of the Census, 3n4
U.S. Chamber of Commerce survey, 9
U.S. Department of Defense (DoD)
  health care system, 65
U.S. Department of Health, Education,
  and Welfare, 59
U.S. Department of Veterans' Affairs,
  65
U.S. Marine Service, 38
  See also U.S. Public Health Service
U.S. Public Health Service (PHS), 38,
  39
  expansion during World War II, 59
  funds for hospital construction from,
    60

increase in services and costs
  (1960s), 64–65
United Steelworkers, 56–57
Utah, 149
Utilization reviews, 21

Veterans' Administration medical
  services, 60, 64, 81
  See also U.S. Department of
    Veterans' Affairs
Virginia, 147
Voucher system
  for Medicare beneficiaries, 139–40
  recommended for Medicaid
    recipients, 145
  for VA and Indian Health Service,
    140

Wagner, Robert, 54
Wagner-Murray-Dingell bill (1943), 80
Walker, Michael A., 94n38
Wall Street Journal/NBC News poll
  (1991), 3, 86
Washingtonian survey (1991), 12–13, 16,
  28n80
Washington (state), 147
Washington State Basic Health Plan,
  109, 110–11, 114
Wasley, Terree P., 145n17
Watts, Harry, 101–2
Waxman, Henry, 115
Weeks, Lewis B., 50
Weinberger, Caspar, 82
Welfare capitalism, 46
Welfare services, private, 32, 45–46
  See also Company doctors;
    Uncompensated care
Welling, Kathryn M., 8n13, 13n34
Wesbury, Stuart A., Jr., 99n57, 102–3,
  107
Wilson, Mr. and Mrs. Luke, 54
Wilson, Woodrow, 39, 78
Winslow, Ron, 9n22
Wisconsin, 149
Woodworth, John, 39
Wyman, Michael, 97
Wyman, Walter, 39

About the Author

Terree P. Wasley is a Washington-based economic consultant who specializes in health care, the federal budget, and tax issues. She previously worked on Capitol Hill as a congressional aide and as an economist for a Virginia-based research foundation and the Economic Policy Division of the U.S. Chamber of Commerce in Washington, D.C.

Wasley received her master's degree in economics from the International College in California. Her economic analyses have been published by the Heritage Foundation and the National Chamber Foundation, as well as numerous magazines and newspapers.

Cato Institute

Founded in 1977, the Cato Institute is a public policy research foundation dedicated to broadening the parameters of policy debate to allow consideration of more options that are consistent with the traditional American principles of limited government, individual liberty, and peace. To that end, the Institute strives to achieve greater involvement of the intelligent, concerned lay public in questions of policy and the proper role of government.

The Institute is named for *Cato's Letters*, libertarian pamphlets that were widely read in the American Colonies in the early 18th century and played a major role in laying the philosophical foundation for the American Revolution.

Despite the achievement of the nation's Founders, today virtually no aspect of life is free from government encroachment. A pervasive intolerance for individual rights is shown by government's arbitrary intrusions into private economic transactions and its disregard for civil liberties.

To counter that trend, the Cato Institute undertakes an extensive publications program that addresses the complete spectrum of policy issues. Books, monographs, and shorter studies are commissioned to examine the federal budget, Social Security, regulation, military spending, international trade, and myriad other issues. Major policy conferences are held throughout the year, from which papers are published thrice yearly in the *Cato Journal*. The Institute also publishes the quarterly magazine *Regulation* and produces a monthly audiotape series, "Perspectives on Policy."

In order to maintain its independence, the Cato Institute accepts no government funding. Contributions are received from foundations, corporations, and individuals, and other revenue is generated from the sale of publications. The Institute is a nonprofit, tax-exempt, educational foundation under Section 501(c)3 of the Internal Revenue Code.

CATO INSTITUTE
224 Second St., S.E.
Washington, D.C. 20003